FRESH START

Bariatric
Cookbook

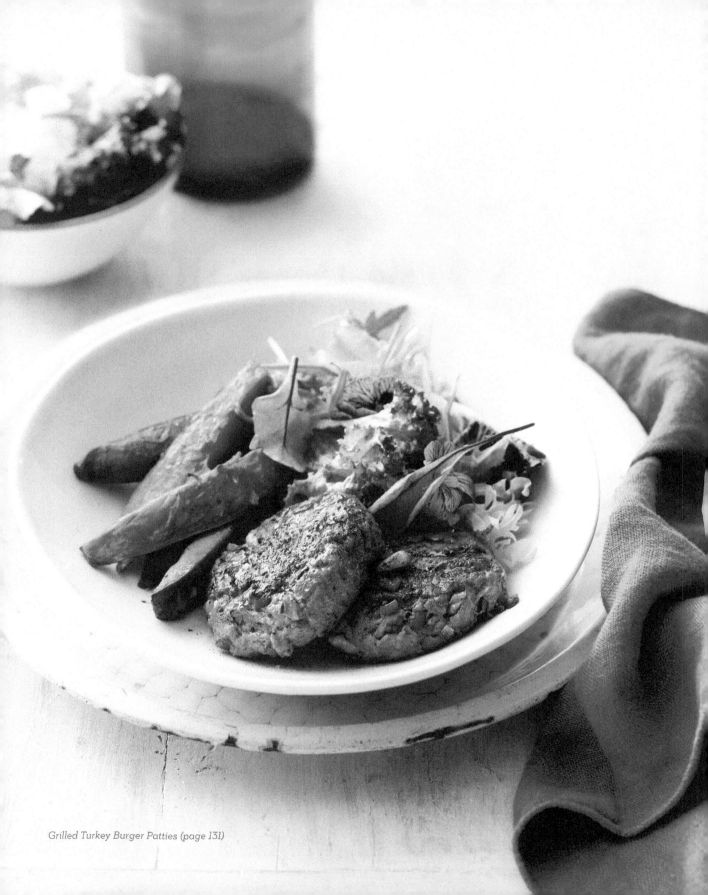

Grilled Turkey Burger Patties (page 131)

FRESH START
Bariatric Cookbook

Healthy Recipes to Enjoy Favorite Foods After Weight-Loss Surgery

SARAH KENT MS, RDN, CD

ROCKRIDGE
PRESS

For my husband,
Christopher

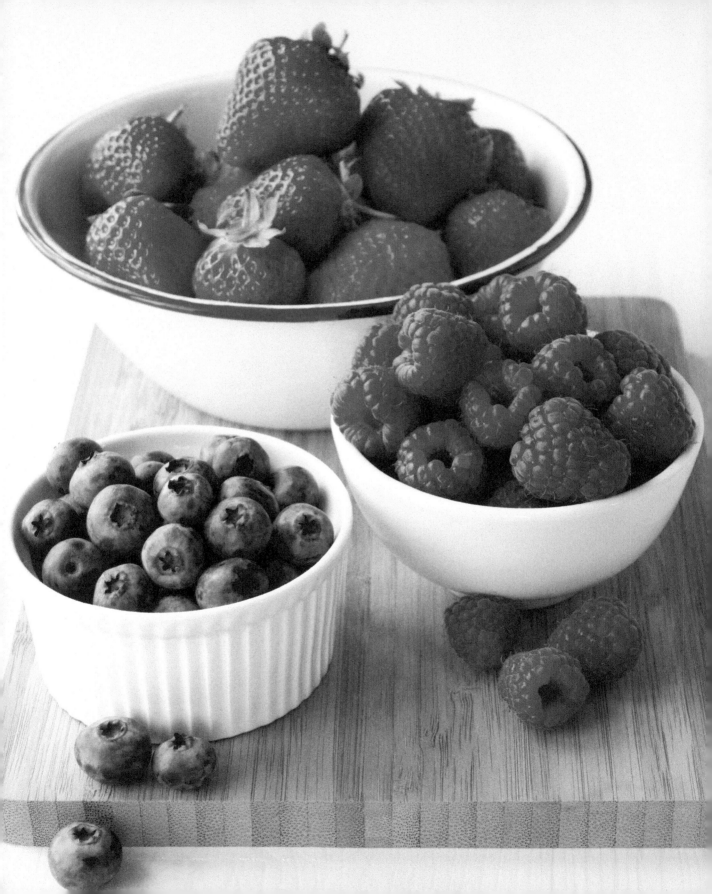

Table of Contents

Introduction

Congratulations, you are ready for this! You have decided to undergo a step—a giant leap, really—away from a life trapped by weight and into a new beginning. Having worked for years as a registered dietitian at an accredited Center of Excellence for bariatric surgery, I can tell you with certainty that there is so much to look forward to. Chasing little ones faster, tying shoes with ease, breathing lighter, taking fewer pills, living longer and stronger—these are just some of the "wins" experienced by my patients who have made permanent lifestyle changes after surgery. But how do you get there and maintain these changes for the long haul, not just for a one-week cleanse or a three-month fad diet?

Your weight-loss journey is a process of changes that take place at both rapid speed and (occasionally) at a snail's pace. The hardest part of the food-related changes—specifically, following a specialized nutrition plan and using the proper ingredients—is committing to them. Probably one of the most daunting realities bariatric surgery patients face is how to establish a new relationship to food and then stick to it. This cookbook is here to ease you into this commitment and make it doable. There's no getting around the fact that commitment is the foundation for long-term success, making your surgery worth it for decades, not just for a year or two.

Now, you might be picking up this book for its many easy and comforting recipes, but there's one very important recipe I want to preview for you here: my recipe not for a particular dish, but for success. There are four core "ingredient skills" that all work together.

1 **Be willing.**

You'll benefit enormously from having the willingness to try something new, or a twist on something familiar. Maybe you haven't tried Greek yogurt yet, but you might find that this creamy, delightful dairy product will satisfy you more than the traditional yogurt cup you ate for years. And did I mention that Greek yogurt has nearly double the protein content?

2 **Make it yours.**

Many fear that they'll have to give up all their favorite foods in return for successful long-term weight loss. This could not be more wrong. By making a few tweaks to the foods you love, you can include most any meal in a long-term post-operative plan.

3 **Be creative.**

You already know that protein is the building block of the bariatric diet, but do not fear—your options range far beyond egg whites and poached fish. Read on to learn tricks for sneaking the all-important protein into a diverse meal plan.

4 **Be resilient.**

Your ability to bounce back after a challenging few days or weeks determines your fate. You are resilient. You *can* live in the present while preparing for the future without preoccupying yourself with the past.

And that's it. You've got it! Mix together these main ingredients to sustain your long-term weight-loss and health goals.

This book starts with *you*, of course, and your surgery team. It's essential that you work closely with the amazing resources available through your surgical center to guide you through this specialized process. I will go through the basic tenets that apply to all, regardless of which particular weight-loss surgery you undergo, but there is no such thing as a cookie-cutter plan. Make sure you consult with a registered dietitian personally to identify specific dietary needs unique to you and your type of surgery.

Now, to the impending question: What's for dinner tonight? How about Baked Fried Chicken Thighs (page 126), mouthwatering Slow Cooker Asian Pork Tenderloin (page 146), or hearty Best-Yet Turkey Chili (page 134)? These are not dishes you once enjoyed but can never have again. Instead, they are easy recipes with tasty flavors and simple ingredients that you can continue to eat while staying straight on your journey to the healthier, stronger, smaller *you!*

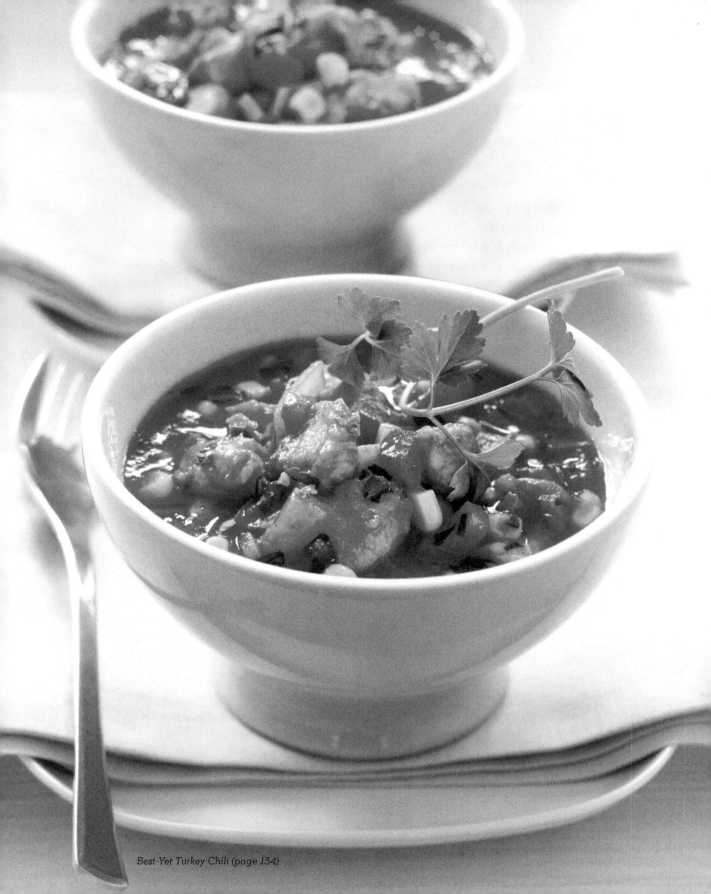

Best-Yet Turkey Chili (page 134)

CHAPTER ONE

Day One and Beyond

The new start on life you've been waiting for is finally here. You may have been preparing for this moment for days, weeks, months, or even years. After surgery, you'll wake up in the same body but excited for the rapid changes that will occur starting nearly immediately. In some ways, it's like Christmas morning: You can't wait to unwrap the gift of weight loss and improved health. In other ways, you're scared: Will you be a success story? This book is designed to help alleviate your fears and answer your questions. It is a guide for eating post-operatively, with plenty of tools to keep you on track, even after any slips along the way. With this information, you will be able to build new habits and grow in confidence. And confidence breeds success.

The Right Decision

Most patients agree that deciding to have bariatric surgery was one of the biggest decisions of their lives. Most patients also agree that, whether solicited or not, opinions about their decision are offered by many people in their lives. Rest assured that no matter what anyone else has said to you, you can wipe away self-doubt. You've made a decision for your health and your life; this is not elective or optional—it is necessary for you.

This decision is supported by a team of highly qualified medical professionals who advise patients using evidence-based research. That means the medical recommendations are based on precedent and scientific outcomes that indicate that the benefits of pursuing a particular path far outweigh the potential risks. So keep pushing forward, and those benefits will appear one by one, and sometimes many all at once. Never doubt that you made the right decision.

Is Enjoying Food Really Possible?

During the first few days post-op, when what you're feasting on is mostly liquid, it's hard to imagine you'll ever find delight in eating food again. Initially, eating may become a chore, something done out of necessity. It's easy for thoughts of the flavors and enjoyment of food to go out the window as you repeatedly think "Gotta get my protein in, need to drink more water . . ." Questions may start to flutter in your head: Will I look forward to eating again? Will I ever be able to eat the foods I used to love?

Keep in mind that right after surgery, your body rapidly undergoes a myriad of physical and hormonal changes—all of which suppress your urge to eat and the amount you are able to eat. Most of your initial rapid weight loss is a product of the combination of these changes. Be patient. As time progresses you will be able to eat a slightly larger volume of food, tolerate a greater variety of food, and have an interest in eating more food.

The good news is that after the first few months, you'll have set a foundation of eating and exercise habits that will sustain your weight loss as time progresses. I know this may sound crazy, but some people who really craved burgers and fries before surgery find that the desire for those types of foods goes away for good. As you transition to eating a diet full of nutritious foods and leave behind high-fat, high-sugar, high-sodium foods, you'll find that your body begins to crave the healthier foods more. And that's the perfect time to try some of your old favorite recipes—with a healthier twist. If you love to cook, it's an opportunity to experiment with spices and seasonings to ensure variety with your protein choices and introduce your family to this new lifestyle.

If you have never spent much time in the kitchen, there are plenty of quick, inexpensive ways to eat nutritiously without a lot of time and fuss. Food is nourishment for your body; it's a necessity to eat every single day. But mealtime is so much more than just what we put in our bodies. It's sitting together for a family dinner, having a candlelit meal to celebrate an anniversary, meeting new people at a church picnic, or reminiscing about what Grandma used to make. The environment in which you choose to eat is just as important as the food in making eating enjoyable. With a little bit of time, some patience, and a willingness to experiment, you can make enjoying nutritious foods truly possible after surgery.

A Cookbook for All Weight-Loss Surgeries

This cookbook is for you. Each recipe has been carefully crafted to meet the needs of patients who have had Roux-en-Y gastric bypass, sleeve gastrectomy, laparoscopic adjustable gastric band placement, or biliopancreatic diversion with duodenal switch (BPD/DS). The diet recommendations in no way replace the recommendations from your medical team but rather serve as a reference summarized from guidelines based on research from the American Society of Metabolic and Bariatric Surgery and the Academy of Nutrition and Dietetics. Each surgery truly is different, and moreover, each person is unique in his or her eating experiences after surgery. There is no one-size-fits-all meal plan.

Use this book as a general guide for how to approach eating, food choice and amounts, and cooking post-operatively with a goal of meeting your weight-loss and nutrition goals—and still enjoying tasty meals. The diet recommendations for each surgery post-op are nearly identical, with a few exceptions you will see frequently noted through this chapter. Note as well the tips at the end of each recipe, which will give more specific guidelines about the timing for when to incorporate each unique recipe into your lifestyle. Take this book with you when you consult with your medical team to serve as a resource for planning meals or anticipating changes in texture in your diet.

TO TELL OR NOT TO TELL

"Wow, you look great! *What* have you been doing to lose all that weight? I have to try it. Tell me all the details!"

You certainly can't keep it a secret that you've lost half of your body weight in less than a year. But do you reveal the intimate details of exactly how this dramatic change came about? What you decide is a personal choice, without a wrong or right answer. It comes down to whatever is most comfortable for you.

Inevitably, you will share the news with some people, whom I put into three groups: supporters, critics, and relaters.

Supporters: You need love, support, encouragement, cheerleading, and coaching. Surgery is not like any diet you've done in the past. If you don't tell anyone what you're going through, it can be more difficult for people to support you through this process. When others have an understanding of the challenges you face, they can learn how you prefer to receive support and encouragement. When your colleagues know you can't have ice cream because you literally *can't* have it, they might be more likely to offer healthier options at the next work picnic. When your great aunt knows you can't eat more than a cup of food, she might be less likely to push the second serving of mashed potatoes during Thanksgiving dinner.

Critics: These are the people who suddenly seem to think they're weight-loss experts and are extremely opinionated about surgery. Their critical response is likely due to lack of knowledge or education about bariatric surgery, their own personal struggle with weight, jealousy, or sheer ignorance. You need to accept that their reaction does not take away from your ability to achieve success after surgery, nor does it validate their response. Again, confidence is key. Your self-worth is not determined by other people's opinions of bariatric surgery.

Relaters: Bariatric surgery is the most successful long-term treatment for obesity—hands down. Unfortunately, many physicians fail to recommend this as an option for appropriate patients, and it's still often falsely viewed as a taboo treatment. According to the Centers for Disease Control and Prevention (CDC), two-thirds of people in the United States are obese or overweight. As someone who's had weight-loss surgery, you can be an inspiration to others and motivate them to take their health back into their own hands. While they won't all have bariatric surgery, they may follow your lead on making healthier lifestyle changes. And you may gain a workout buddy, a farmers' market friend, or a willing ear to talk with along the way.

Bariatric Nutritional Know-How

By the time most people undergo bariatric surgery, they are quite familiar with common weight-loss diets. The thought of memorizing the ins and outs of yet another eating plan is more than cringeworthy for many people. Fortunately, what you've already learned about following diets in the past will serve as a foundation for learning how to eat after bariatric surgery. You don't need to be a nutrition expert to understand and follow a bariatric eating plan. Let's review the principles for eating after surgery, which are represented throughout the recipes in this cookbook.

Liquids

Staying hydrated after surgery is the first and most important rule. Drinking enough liquids will not only increase your energy, but it will also help significantly with your weight loss. Additionally, dehydration is the most common complication of surgery, and one that can easily be prevented. It can be challenging at first, partly because there is no drinking with meals or 30 minutes before or after eating. Be proactive and always carry a beverage with you. Focus on drinking throughout the day and evening to prevent trying to catch up later—your small pouch will prohibit you from chugging large amounts of fluid at one time.

- ▶ **What to Drink:** water, milk, soy milk, protein shakes, decaffeinated tea or coffee (without added cream or sugar), and any other noncarbonated and sugar-free beverages (sweetened with sugar substitutes is okay)
- ▶ **Amount per Day:** 64 to 100 ounces—progressing in volume throughout your post-op diet stages
- ▶ **What to Limit or Avoid:** juices, caffeinated beverages (including soda, coffee, tea, and energy drinks), carbonated waters, alcohol, lemonade, sweetened tea, sugary sports drinks, and any sugar-sweetened beverages

Protein

It's all about protein, the most important macronutrient to take in post-operatively. Protein is the building block of muscle and tissue. It's crucial to eat adequate protein while following a very low-calorie diet. When you eat enough protein, you will feel energized, lose more fat while preserving muscle, and experience longer post-meal satisfaction. Protein is digested more slowly than carbohydrates and contains fewer calories than fats. Initially post-op, you will take in only water and protein-rich foods. As you progress, you will slowly add more mixed meals into your diet. This cookbook is essential to give you a variety of ideas for eating adequate protein for the long haul so meals don't become boring. Eating protein at every meal for a lifetime is essential to not only lose weight and heal initially but to maintain weight loss for the long term.

▶ **What to Eat:** eggs, poultry (chicken and turkey without skin, lean nitrate-free chicken or turkey sausage, ground chicken, and turkey breast), all fish and seafood, low-fat dairy products (low-fat Greek yogurt, 1 percent or nonfat cottage cheese, and 1 percent or nonfat milk and cheese), lean beef (if tolerated, beginning 3 months post-op; sirloin, loin, round roast or steak, and lean or supreme lean ground beef), lean pork (if tolerated, beginning 3 months post-op; tenderloin, top loin chop, and ham with visible fat removed), and vegetarian protein sources (beans, nuts, lentils, and seeds)

▶ **Amount per Day:** 60 to 100 grams (Note: Specific recommendations are based on ideal body weight and the post-operative diet stage.)

▶ **What to Limit or Avoid:** high-fat dairy products (cream and whole milk), high-fat cuts of beef or pork (pork sausage, bacon, bologna, salami, pork ribs, and ground beef), and skin-on poultry

PROTEIN SOURCE	PORTION SIZE	PROTEIN (GRAMS)*
Poultry, beef, pork, fish	2 ounces	14 grams (7 grams per ounce)
Shrimp, scallops	3 ounces (about 15 large)	18 grams
Lunch meat (turkey, chicken, ham, or roast beef)	2 ounces (4 to 6 thin slices)	10 grams
Egg	1 large	6 to 7 grams
Egg whites	2 large	8 grams
Cottage or ricotta cheese (1% to 2% fat)	½ cup	14 grams
Natural cheese (Cheddar, Colby, mozzarella, Swiss, etc.)	1 ounce or 1 slice	7 grams
Greek yogurt	6 ounces (¾ cup)	10 to 15 grams
Yogurt	6 ounces (¾ cup)	5 grams
Lentils	½ cup cooked	9 grams
Beans	½ cup cooked	5 to 9 grams

Individual protein content may vary; always check the nutrition facts label.

DRINKING YOUR PROTEIN

There's no escaping a protein drink during the first few days and weeks after surgery. Getting enough protein is a full-time job, and without allowing some liquid sources, it may be nearly impossible. On the other hand, we want to set a solid eating plan for the long term since you aren't going to drink protein shakes for breakfast, lunch, and dinner the rest of your life. I favor a plan where the pureed diet is introduced early after surgery to include whole foods. In between meals, milk is an acceptable alternative to commercial protein shakes (see High-Protein Milk, page 30). Carefully focus on eating only high-quality protein foods in the first few weeks post-op since it's difficult to get in large volumes of food. Don't forget, you actually *burn* more calories digesting whole foods than liquids. So reconsider trying pureed turkey chili! Here are some recommendations for bariatric-friendly protein powders:

- ▶ **Choose whey protein isolate.** It's easiest for your body to absorb and is the most dense in essential amino acids. Try the brands biPro or UNJURY.
- ▶ **Other high-quality sources:** Two of these are soy protein isolate (vegan) and egg white powder.
- ▶ **Try an unflavored version.** These are low in calories and clean, being free from artificial ingredients.
- ▶ **Tips for flavored versions**: Choose varieties that are completely sugar-free and sweetened with stevia, sucralose (Splenda), or other sugar substitutes. There are hundreds of options, from vanilla to butter pecan, which will leave you satisfied for very few calories. Sugar substitutes are FDA approved, calorie-free, safe to have after surgery, and not linked to dumping syndrome. Be cautious with sugar alcohols (erythritol, mannitol, xylitol, and sorbitol), as they contribute some calories and can cause unpleasant gastrointestinal side effects.

Carbohydrates

A quick source of energy for your body, including your brain, carbohydrates are important for many metabolic functions. During the initial post-operative diet, you will take in little to no carbs. Your body will function normally by obtaining energy from metabolizing fat stores and using protein from the foods you are eating. Carbohydrates can be found in two varieties: simple or complex. Simple carbohydrates are digested quickly, and easily turn into sugar in our blood, giving us a quick energy rush and a subsequent crash. Simple carbs include foods made with white refined flour, candies, sodas, juice drinks, and many processed foods.

Complex carbohydrates are digested more slowly and are rich in fiber, vitamins, and minerals. They include 100 percent whole-grain foods, fruits, and vegetables. Focus on limiting simple carbs and eating more complex carbs.

► **What to Eat:** fresh fruits, vegetables, sweet potatoes or white potatoes with skin, oatmeal, 100 percent whole-grain products (toasted are better tolerated than doughy fresh), brown or wild rice or 100 percent whole-wheat pasta (if tolerated), barley and ancient grains (quinoa, spelt, farrow, and millet)

► **Amount per Day:** very small amounts initially; after the first year and long term, aim for no more than 35 to 45 percent of total calories from carbohydrates

► **What to Limit or Avoid:** any white refined grain products (white bread, white pasta, and crackers), cookies, candies, cakes, pastries, juices (including fruit juice), sodas, and chips

A NOTE ABOUT SUGAR

Simple sugars are not tolerated after surgery. Dumping syndrome is a condition that can occur after eating foods high in sugar and, in some cases, eating too many carbohydrates at one time. Symptoms occur shortly after consuming the food in question and include some combination of feeling shaky, lightheaded, sweaty, or dizzy (with a possibility of fainting), increased heart rate, drop in blood sugar (reactive hypoglycemia), abdominal cramping, and diarrhea. People who have had the Roux-en-Y gastric bypass or BPD/DS are most at risk for experiencing dumping syndrome. Those who have had the sleeve gastrectomy also may experience this side effect as well. Avoid this uncomfortable condition by completely avoiding foods high in sugar. A general recommendation is to avoid processed foods with more than 10 to 15 grams of sugar per serving. Remember, you are encouraged to eat whole fruits and dairy products, both of which contain some natural sugars.

Fats

Dietary fats are important to absorb essential fat-soluble vitamins—A, D, E, and K. Additionally, there are some essential fatty acids (omega-3s and omega-6s) our bodies cannot make and must ingest instead. Fats are the most calorie-dense of all macronutrients at 9 calories per gram, so we must always be careful of portion sizes—even in the healthy versions. Be cautious with processed foods labeled as fat-free or low fat, as they often replace fat with more sugar or sodium to improve the flavor of the food. Dairy products, particularly milk, yogurt, and cottage cheese, should be eaten in low-fat or nonfat form to save on calories and artery-clogging saturated fats. Choose these versions when cooking as often as possible. Note that nonfat or 1 percent milk does not contain any fewer vitamins, minerals, or grams of protein compared to whole milk. Choose full-fat foods in the form of vegetable oils, nuts, seeds, avocados, olives, and fatty fish—all of which are heart healthy.

▶ **What to Eat:** avocados, canola oil, chia seeds, fatty fish (salmon, mackerel, and tuna), seafood, flaxseed, olive oil, almonds, walnuts, peanuts, and all-natural nut butters

▶ **Amount per Day:** very limited amounts initially; long term, no more than 30 percent of total calories from fats (mostly monounsaturated and polyunsaturated fats and less than 7 percent from saturated fats)

▶ **What to Limit:** butter, tropical oils (palm and coconut oil), full-fat dairy, and miscellaneous vegetable oils

▶ **What to Avoid:** animal fats (fat on meats, lard), fried foods, stick margarines containing trans fats, and foods high in saturated fats

Vitamin and Mineral Supplements

Food is the best source of the nutrients your body needs after bariatric surgery, but due to the restricted amount of food you are able to eat and changes in the absorption of certain nutrients, all bariatric surgery patients need to be on vitamin and mineral supplements post-op. Follow the recommendations from your bariatric surgery team for specific details. Here is some information on common vitamin and mineral supplements:

▶ **Multivitamin with minerals,** whether in chewable or liquid form, is required for all, regardless of which surgery you have. Make sure the vitamins and minerals come to 100 to 200 percent of daily recommended values.

▶ **Vitamin D** is advised for most everyone, since nearly all who qualify for the surgery tend to be deficient in it.

▶ **Calcium** is recommended for almost all patients post-operatively due to the importance of bone health.

▶ **Iron** is often recommend especially after the Roux-en-Y gastric bypass or BPD/DS, since changes after these surgeries make it difficult for the body to absorb iron.

▶ **Vitamin B$_{12}$** is advised, especially after the Roux-en-Y gastric bypass or BPD/DS and potentially with the sleeve gastrectomy. It is important for proper nerve function and for preventing anemia.

- **Certain fat-soluble vitamins,** to be discussed with your team, are recommended after the BPD/DS.
- **B-complex** provides additional B-vitamin supplementation and may be recommended after any type of bariatric surgery. It contains high doses of thiamine, which is important for metabolism.

Bottom line: Due to the nature of these surgeries, taking certain vitamin and mineral supplements is a commitment for life. I have seen deficiencies appear several years down the road when people reached their goal weight and stopped taking their supplements. Make sure to follow up regularly with your medical team to have your blood levels of these important nutrients tested.

Equipment

You will find that the majority of the recipes in this book require very little more than a cutting board, sauté pan, and a good knife! Here are a few must-have tools to have in your kitchen to help you prepare some of the recipes in this cookbook. You can easily find most of them at major department stores for a reasonable price.

Immersion or hand blender Use for pureeing soups, chilies, or other dishes while they're still on the stove.

Mini blender or food processor (dishwasher safe) Puree small portions of foods for yourself or make a single-serving shake.

Mini muffin tin These are great for portion control.

Slow cooker The 5-quart size is sufficient for the recipes in this book, but you may opt for smaller or larger versions.

Spiralizer Use for making zucchini noodles in place of pasta; try the small handheld versions.

Vegetable peeler Use for removing tough skins of fruits and vegetables that aren't tolerated in the first few months post-op.

QUIETING SELF-JUDGMENTS

We all know the phrase "You are what you eat," but try this one: "You are what you believe." How much do your thoughts, feelings, and judgments impact your behaviors and overall state of well-being? In short, a lot. The practice of mindfulness is growing in popularity because it emphasizes awareness and acceptance of the present moment. By staying in the moment, we can focus on what we are doing, rather than chastise ourselves for past mistakes, regrets, and negative feelings. And when we start to judge ourselves, which is inevitable, a short mindfulness exercise can quickly take us out of it. Here are two mindfulness exercises to help us stay in the moment and recognize and be grateful for the good things we have.

Mindful eating

1 *Eat at a table without distractions.* That's right, turn off the TV and put your smartphone or tablet somewhere else. Notice the time that you start eating your meal. Take a bite of food, and chew 20 to 30 times before swallowing.

2 *Put down your fork in between bites.* Savor the flavor and the consistency: Is it savory, sweet, sour, or salty? Repeat these steps until your plate is half empty. Notice the clock again. Have 10 to 15 minutes gone by? If not, slow down and wait.

3 *Engage in conversation or take a few deep breaths.* Aim for 30 minutes to eat your entire meal. Clean off the kitchen table and put flowers, decorative placements, and perhaps even candles on it to remind you that mealtime is meant to be both enjoyable and relaxing.

Gratitude

1 *Use snail mail more often.* Write out a thank-you card and send it to your walking buddy. Dedicate a small amount of time per week to write out recognition for work colleagues.

2 *Keep a daily personal journal.* Focus on writing down the best part of your day, every day. Expressing gratitude for the people in our lives may help us experience compassion for ourselves. Start focusing on creating positive thoughts, and watch them multiply!

Texture Week by Week

Diet progression should be guided by your individual bariatric team; however, here is a list of general guidelines.

SLEEVE GASTRECTOMY, ROUX-EN-Y GASTRIC BYPASS

BPD/DS also generally follows these same guidelines

Post-operative Timeline	Diet Type
Days 1 to 2	Clear liquid diet
Weeks 1 to 2	(FL) Full liquid diet
Week 3	(P) Pureed foods
Weeks 4 to 6	(S) Soft foods
Week 7 or 8+	(G) Advance to general foods

LAPAROSCOPIC ADJUSTABLE GASTRIC BAND

Post-operative Timeline	Diet Type
Days 1 to 2	Clear liquid diet
Weeks 1 to 2	(FL) Full liquid diet
Week 3	(P) Pureed foods
Week 4	(S) Soft foods
Week 5 or 6+	(G) Advance to general foods
Following a fill or adjustment	Full liquid diet for 2 to 3 days. Advance to pureed foods for 2 to 3 days and then soft foods for 3 to 4 days as tolerated. Gradually progress to general foods.

The Bariatric Kitchen

Your kitchen is your workshop after surgery. Fortunately, you don't need a complete kitchen makeover to eat well after surgery. You just need a few important staples and pieces of equipment to prepare fast, delicious meals and ensure that you will have long-term weight-loss success.

Toss It	Stock Up
Vegetable oil	Extra-virgin olive oil
All-purpose flour	Whole-wheat pastry flour
Sour cream	Low-fat plain Greek yogurt, hummus
Processed cheeses and cheese spreads	Natural cheeses (mozzarella, Cheddar, Feta, etc.), cottage cheese
Canned premade soups	Canned or dried beans for making homemade soups, low-sodium broth
Hot dogs, bacon	100% natural nitrate-free chicken or turkey sausage
Instant oatmeal packets	100% old-fashioned rolled oats or steel-cut oats, unsweetened
Fruit snacks	Fresh fruits, 100% natural (unsweetened) applesauce
Salami, bologna, pastrami	Deli-sliced (nitrate-free) turkey, chicken, lean roast beef
Juice	Fresh lemons and limes, sliced, for water, herbal tea
Potato chips and pretzels	Dehydrated vegetables/snap peas (Snapea Crisps or Lentil Snaps), kale chips
Flavored regular yogurt	Plain yogurt, low-sugar Greek yogurt
Canned high-fat meats	Canned chicken breast, packets or cans of tuna or salmon
Pasta	Fresh spaghetti squash and spiralized zucchini instead of pasta
Creamy processed salad dressings	Flavored vinegars and olive oil

Tips for Success

The following recommendations for after surgery are here to help you make sure you not only get down to your goal weight but keep it off. These are tried-and-true tips based on my experience in working with successful post-op bariatric surgery patients who are more than five years out from surgery.

Dedicate yourself to your bariatric clinic for life.
The specialists in the field know what to look for to make sure you maintain your healthy lifestyle and avoid long-term complications. A quick fix found in the bariatric clinic is something that could be easily missed by a primary care physician.

Just walk.
It's easy to stop exercising when the pounds just fall off during the first few months after surgery. Walking seems so simple—but it's the most common exercise done regularly by post-op patients for the long term. So lace up your shoes and head out.

Don't skimp on your protein. Ever.
A few years out from surgery, it might be tempting to go back to cereal for breakfast and a sandwich for lunch with little in between the bread. But when you are tempted to nosh nearly 30 minutes later, you might see the pounds start to pack back on. Focus on making half of your meals protein for the long term and balancing the rest with other foods to keep you interested.

Fluid load.
Filling up on plenty of water before and in between meals is a sure-fire trick to avoid mindless snacking and overeating at mealtimes. Get yourself a favorite water bottle and make it a priority to get in 100 ounces or more per day long term. After six months post-op, try fluid-loading to help reduce the amount of food you are able to eat at a meal. Continue avoiding fluids during and after the meal, but within 10 minutes of starting a meal, slam a glass of water. It may actually help you feel more full and eat less. Keep in mind that drinking 10 minutes—instead of 30 minutes—before a meal is only advised for when you're six months post-op.

Find a bariatric surgery support group.
Your journey doesn't end when you hit your goal weight; get yourself connected with a support group to establish a network of people for lifelong support. You may need a listening ear or you may be an inspiration to others.

FOODS TO AVOID AFTER SURGERY

The long-term post-op goal is to live a normal life, eating most foods in moderation. A big fear for patients is getting sick (dumping syndrome, abdominal discomfort, or vomiting) after surgery. During the first three months after surgery, some foods should be avoided completely to prevent these scenarios from occurring, but many foods can be slowly added back over time as your body adjusts to its "new" stomach.

Laparoscopic Adjustable Gastric Band

Liquids Carbonated beverages, alcohol, caffeinated beverages

Proteins Dry, tough meat, poultry, or fish

Carbohydrates Rice, pasta, doughy bread products (untoasted breads); dried fruits, skin-on fruit, fresh pineapple; popcorn; dry fibrous cereals such as granola and bran cereal

Fats Raw nuts and seeds, fried foods, greasy foods (skin-on poultry, fat on meat), peanut butter and nut butters (sticky)

Other Foods Coconut, asparagus stalks, rubbery microwaved or reheated foods (due to texture)

Sleeve Gastrectomy, Roux-en-Y Gastric Bypass, and BPD/DS

Liquids Carbonated beverages, alcohol, caffeinated beverages, fruit juices, any sugary beverages

Proteins Dry, tough meat, poultry, or fish

Carbohydrates Rice, pasta, doughy bread products (untoasted breads); dried fruits, skin-on fruit, fresh pineapple; popcorn; dry fibrous cereals such as granola and bran cereal

Fats Raw nuts and seeds, fried foods, greasy foods (skin-on poultry, fat on meat), peanut butter and nut butters (sticky)

Other Foods Asparagus stalks, raw celery, coconut, sugar-sweetened sauces and condiments, cookies, candy

This Book's Recipes

The recipes in this book are a mix of simple, familiar meals with a healthy twist and a few foodie favorites. Home at 5:00 p.m. and need dinner by 6:00 p.m.? No problem! Most of these meals can be made in 30 minutes, and many are slow cooker meals that are table ready when you walk in the door. Notice the servings yield for each recipe—many produce big portions intentionally, so you can serve your family and have leftovers for meals later in the week. Nutrition facts are listed for each recipe, including grams of protein, carbohydrates, and sugars. Be aware that while the nutrition facts are listed per serving size, your individual portion size may vary, so you may need to adjust accordingly. I've also included recommended servings based on which dietary stage you're in post-op. Look for these icons in the recipes:

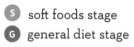

FL full liquid stage   **S** soft foods stage

P puree stage   **G** general diet stage

Focus, too, on the recipe tips, which give ideas about how to enjoy each recipe throughout the stages of your diet post-op.

You will also see some recipes for snacks and desserts. Mindless snacking results in unnecessary calories and should be avoided. Focus instead on eating three meals a day and drinking liquids in between meals (including milk or protein shakes). Cautiously eat snacks in between meals, and monitor portions closely. As for desserts, these recipes give you an idea of what to bring to the family picnic or share at a birthday party so that you can enjoy the festivities without getting sick from typical high-sugar, high-fat desserts. These should be enjoyed on special occasions and not as part of your daily diet. Although these recipes are all appropriate for after surgery, you still need to be cautious of extra calories that can add up quickly.

A few basic reminders:

▶ Eat slowly—aim to take 30 minutes to eat a meal.

▶ Avoid drinking with meals or for 30 minutes before or after a meal.

▶ Take your essential vitamin and mineral supplements.

▶ Avoid grazing or mindless snacking.

▶ Be active every day.

▶ Always eat protein-rich foods *first*.

Eating Well for Life

You have all the ingredients to achieve your successful weight-loss recipe. The one last concern on your mind may be your lifelong relationship with food—and in many cases it's a struggle. But you can rebuild that relationship; you can retrain your brain to avoid falling into old habits. Start by setting small, achievable goals— weekly, if possible. Congratulate yourself on your progress, but don't criticize yourself if you don't achieve a goal. Just keep setting new ones. Bariatric surgery truly is a lifelong journey. Do your best to honor your promises to eat health- fully and stay active, and you will be able to maintain your healthier lifestyle for decades to come.

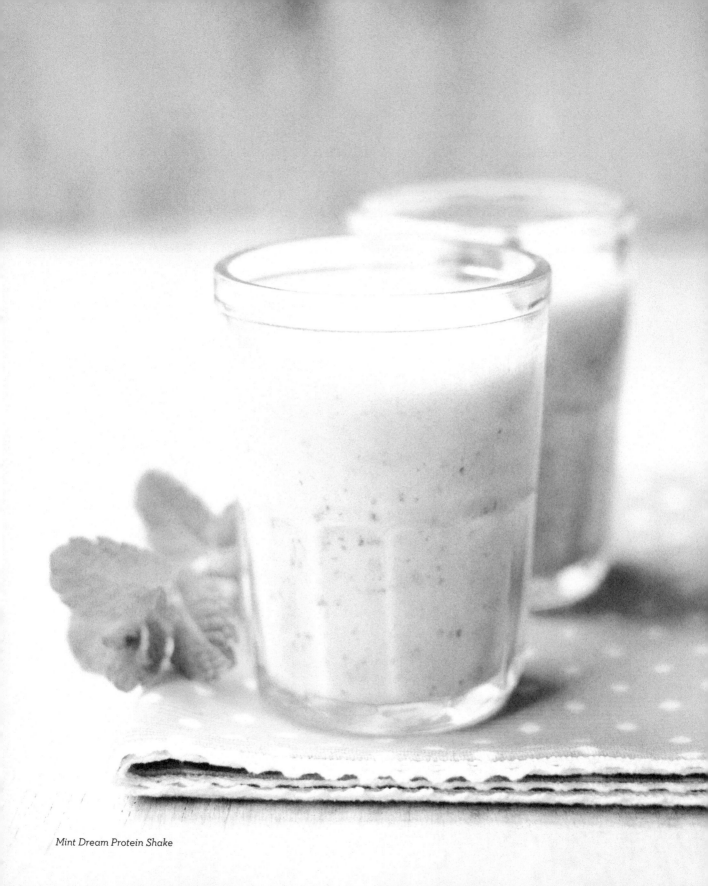

Mint Dream Protein Shake

Early Post-Op Foods

High-Protein Milk

MAKES 4 SERVINGS / PREP: 5 MINUTES / TOTAL: 5 MINUTES

You don't have to spend a lot of money on expensive protein powders to make sure you drink enough liquid protein. You might think this recipe is too simple, but it's here to remind you that drinking your protein doesn't have to be complicated and costly. Try this milk as an alternative to a protein shake, or use it in place of milk in any recipe that calls for some. It'll cost you only about 40 cents per cup to make, and it brings a whopping 14 grams of protein!

4 cups skim milk

1 cup nonfat dry milk powder

Post-Op Servings

FL 1 cup, as many times per day as needed to reach protein goal

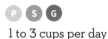

1 to 3 cups per day

1 In a deep bowl or a blender, beat the milk and milk powder slowly with a beater or blend on high speed to mix for about 5 minutes, until the powder is well dissolved and no longer visible.

2 Refrigerate any milk you don't drink or use right away. The flavor improves overnight. Discard any remaining milk after 7 days.

Did you know? *Milk is an excellent source of protein for immediately after surgery, as well as for the long term. All cow's milk contains at least 8 grams of protein per cup with varied fat and calorie content. Consider trying a brand such as Fairlife, which produces milk that contains fewer carbohydrates and more protein per cup. Keep in mind that both cow's milk and nonfat milk powder contain lactose, the natural sugar found in milk. For individuals who may be lactose intolerant, lactose-free milk or soy milk is a well-tolerated, appropriate alternative. Be aware that other plant-based milks such as almond, rice, or coconut milk contain no or extremely low amounts of protein.*

Per Serving (1 cup): Calories: 144 Total fat: 0g Sodium: 218mg
Total carbs: 21g Sugar: 21g Fiber: 0g Protein: 14g

Iced Coffee Protein Shake

SERVES 2 / PREP TIME: 5 MINUTES / TOTAL TIME: 5 MINUTES

Do they know you by name at your local Starbucks? Are you struggling with giving up your favorite cup of java in the morning? It's true that most dietitians would approve of drinking a cup of black decaffeinated coffee after surgery (no added cream or sugars, of course). But until patients have a good handle on the post-operative diet and drinking enough water, it's recommended that you pass on caffeine and permanently eliminate any sugary high-calorie coffee drinks. The good news is that you can still get your coffee flavor fix with this protein shake.

1 scoop (¼ cup) vanilla
   protein powder
1 cup decaffeinated coffee,
   brewed and chilled
1 cup low-fat milk
½ teaspoon cinnamon
½ cup ice

1 In a blender, pour the milk, then add the protein powder, cinnamon, and ice. Blend on high speed, about 3 to 4 minutes, until the shake is smooth and the protein powder is well dissolved.

2 Refrigerate any shake you don't drink or use right away, and reblend prior to serving. Discard any remaining shake after 7 days.

Per serving: Calories: 102 Total fat: 0g Sodium: 155 mg
Total Carbs: 8g Sugar: 6g Fiber: 0g Protein: 14g

Post-Op Servings

FL 1 cup, as many times per day as needed to reach protein goal

P S G

1 to 3 cups per day

Chocolate Lovers' Protein Shake

MAKES 2 SERVINGS / PREP: 5 MINUTES / TOTAL: 5 MINUTES

Chocolate is an all-time favorite sweet treat. Even a small bite can start to produce some of the feel-good endorphins, like serotonin, in our brain. Fortunately, there is a way to meet your chocolate fix without the extra sugar found in most chocolate treats. Whip up this shake with chocolate flavor from both the protein powder and cocoa powder, and you will be in chocolate lovers' heaven.

1 cup low-fat milk

½ cup low-fat
   cottage cheese

1 scoop (¼ cup) chocolate
   or plain protein powder

2 tablespoons
   unsweetened
   cocoa powder

½ teaspoon vanilla extract

5 ice cubes

Post-Op Servings

FL P S G

1 to 3 cups per day

1 In a blender, blend on high speed to combine the milk, cottage cheese, protein powder, cocoa powder, vanilla, and ice for 2 to 3 minutes, until the shake is smooth and the powders are well dissolved.

2 Pour half the shake into a glass and enjoy.

3 Refrigerate any shake you don't drink or use right away, and reblend prior to serving. Discard any remaining shake after 7 days.

Did you know? *Chocolate is made from the cocoa, or cacao, bean, which is loaded with heart-healthy antioxidants and protective flavonols. Unfortunately, most chocolate in desserts is loaded with added fats and sugar and has little of the true cocoa bean. Using 100 percent unsweetened cocoa powder, you can make low-sugar desserts and treats, or try simply mixing it with milk to get the antioxidant and chocolate fix without the sugar.*

Per Serving: Calories: 188 Total fat: 5g Sodium: 38mg Total carbs: 14g Sugar: 3g Fiber: 2g Protein: 25g

Mint Dream Protein Shake

MAKES 2 SERVINGS / PREP: 5 MINUTES / TOTAL: 5 MINUTES

Take me back to the 1950s, when ice cream drinks were all the rage. A meal wasn't complete unless it was capped off with a cool, creamy dessert like a Grasshopper: a combination of sweet chocolate, vanilla ice cream, and mint liqueur. Try this (yes, alcohol-free) Mint Dream Shake as a perfectly delightful substitute. Toss in the secret ingredient, a handful of fresh spinach, to give this shake some extra green, and you will never even know it's there! Enjoy this shake after dinner to satisfy your sweet tooth and finish off your protein goal for the day.

1 small handful (less than 1 cup) fresh spinach

1 cup low-fat milk

1 scoop (¼ cup) vanilla protein powder

¼ cup low-fat plain Greek yogurt

1 tablespoon cocoa powder

½ teaspoon peppermint extract

3 ice cubes

2 to 3 fresh mint sprigs, for garnish

Post-Op Servings

FL P S G

1 to 3 cups per day

1 In a blender, blend on high speed to combine the spinach, milk, protein powder, yogurt, cocoa powder, peppermint extract, and ice for 3 to 4 minutes, until the spinach is thoroughly pureed and the powders are well dissolved.

2 Pour half the shake into a glass, garnish with the fresh mint sprigs, and enjoy.

3 Refrigerate any shake you don't drink or use right away, and reblend prior to serving. Discard any remaining shake after 1 day.

Did you know? *Spinach is an excellent source of iron. After a Roux-en-Y gastric bypass (or BPD), iron absorption is impaired in the body, and many people need to take iron supplements. Toss a handful of spinach into your next protein shake to help you reach your iron needs. Other high-quality sources of iron include meats and beans.*

Per Serving (1 cup): Calories: 135 Total fat: 1g Sodium: 115mg
Total carbs: 12g Sugar: 8g Fiber: 1g Protein: 18g

Dreamsicle Protein Shake

MAKES 2 SERVINGS / PREP: 5 MINUTES / TOTAL: 5 MINUTES

Nothing says refreshing like fresh citrus flavors. Chocolate and vanilla can get boring after a while, so give your taste buds a treat and try something with a sweet orange flavor. This protein shake will give you the creamy orange flavor of an Orange Julius. The cottage cheese is a key ingredient for not only protein but to help give it an ultracreamy texture.

1½ cups ice

½ cup low-fat cottage cheese

½ cup water, plus 2 to 4 tablespoons additional if needed

1 small tangerine or mandarin orange (about 2 ounces) or 1 small mandarin orange fruit cup, drained

1 scoop (¼ cup) unflavored or vanilla protein powder

1 teaspoon powdered stevia extract

½ teaspoon vanilla extract

1 In a blender, blend on high speed to combine the ice, cottage cheese, water, tangerine, protein powder, stevia, and vanilla for 2 to 3 minutes, until the shake is smooth and no longer lumpy. Add 2 to 4 tablespoons more water if the shake is too thick.

2 Pour half the shake into a glass and enjoy.

3 Refrigerate any shake you don't drink or use right away, and reblend prior to serving. Discard any remaining shake after 7 days.

Per Serving (1 cup): Calories: 137 Total fat 1g Sodium: 104mg
Total carbs 12g Sugar: 8g Fiber: 1g Protein: 21g

Post-Op Servings

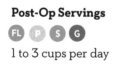

1 to 3 cups per day

Strawberry Crème Protein Shake

MAKES 2 SERVINGS / PREP: 5 MINUTES / TOTAL: 5 MINUTES

Strawberry milk shake on your mind? Save yourself from consuming a day's worth of calories in one drink by trying this version instead. The Greek yogurt gives this shake a creamy texture, just like the one from your local ice cream stand. Using frozen strawberries will keep the mixture extra thick, while fresh berries will make a thinner, more melted version.

1 cup low-fat milk or unsweetened soy milk

1 cup fresh or frozen strawberries

½ cup low-fat plain Greek yogurt

1 scoop (¼ cup) vanilla or unflavored protein powder

½ teaspoon vanilla extract

1 In a blender, blend on high speed to combine the milk, strawberries, yogurt, protein powder, and vanilla for 2 to 3 minutes, until the shake is smooth and the protein powder is well dissolved.

2 Pour half the shake into a glass and enjoy.

3 Refrigerate any shake you don't drink or use right away, and reblend prior to serving. Discard any remaining shake after 7 days.

Per Serving (1 cup): Calories: 145 Total fat: 2g Sodium: 92mg
Total carbs: 15g Sugar: 6g Fiber: 1g Protein: 15g

Post-Op Servings

FL P S G

1 to 3 cups per day

Cherry-Almond Protein Shake

MAKES 2 SERVINGS / PREP: 5 MINUTES / TOTAL: 5 MINUTES

This delicious shake has flavors like the classic cherries jubilee and will satisfy your cravings for a creamy cherries fix. Using frozen fruit not only helps you save on cost, especially during the off-season months, but it will give this shake an even creamier texture. No almond extract in the house? No problem—swap for vanilla extract in a pinch.

1 (5.3-ounce) cup low-fat black cherry yogurt (see tip)

½ cup water

½ cup low-fat milk

¼ cup frozen pitted cherries

1 scoop (¼ cup) vanilla or plain protein powder

½ teaspoon almond extract

Post-Op Servings

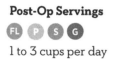

1 to 3 cups per day

1 In a blender, blend on high speed to combine the yogurt, water, milk, cherries, protein powder, and almond extract for 2 to 3 minutes, until the shake is smooth and the protein powder is well dissolved.

2 Pour half the shake into a glass and enjoy.

3 Refrigerate any shake you don't drink or use right away, and reblend prior to serving. Discard any remaining shake after 7 days.

Ingredient tip: *I love the brand siggi's, which makes a delicious low-fat, high-protein black cherry yogurt. If you can't find it, plain Greek yogurt will always have the most protein and lowest sugar content per serving. Choose plain when possible and add in your own flavoring, such as stevia extract, sugar-free fruit preserves, sugar-free pudding mix, cocoa powder, or cinnamon to add flavor without added sugars. When you're on a general post-op diet, add fresh fruit to plain yogurt for sweetness. Read labels carefully to find flavored Greek yogurt options with the lowest amount of sugar possible without missing out on protein. Look for versions with less than 10 grams of sugar and more than 12 grams of protein per serving.*

Per Serving (1 cup): Calories: 158 Total fat: 1g Sodium: 89mg
Total carbs: 16g Sugar: 12g Fiber: 0g Protein: 20g

Chocolate–Peanut Butter Smoothie

MAKES 2 SERVINGS / PREP: 5 MINUTES / TOTAL: 5 MINUTES

Craving a Reese's Peanut Butter Cup or perhaps a chocolate–peanut butter ice cream sundae? Look no further for a low-calorie, low-carb option that will satisfy your urge for peanut butter goodness. This protein smoothie includes the flavors of rich chocolate and creamy peanut butter all mixed into one drink. Craving satisfied!

1 cup low-fat milk

½ cup low-fat plain Greek yogurt

1 scoop (¼ cup) vanilla protein powder

2 tablespoons powdered peanut butter

2 tablespoons cocoa powder

1 In a blender, blend on high speed to combine the milk, yogurt, protein powder, powdered peanut butter, and cocoa powder for 3 to 4 minutes, until the powders are well dissolved and no longer visible.

2 Pour half the smoothie into a glass and enjoy.

3 Refrigerate any smoothie you don't drink or use right away, and reblend prior to serving. Discard any remaining smoothie after 7 days.

Post-Op Servings

FL 1 cup, as many times per day as needed to reach protein goal

P **S** **G**

1 to 3 cups per day

Serving tip: *While this smoothie is excellent for a full liquid diet in the initial days and weeks post-op, it also makes a great supplemental protein source for the long term. Drink it after dinner to accomplish your protein goals, or simply as a delicious substitute for dessert.*

Per Serving: Calories: 185 Total fat: 3g Sodium: 173mg Total carbs: 17g Sugar: 10g Fiber: 3g Protein: 24g

Pumpkin Delight Smoothie

MAKES 2 SERVINGS / PREP: 5 MINUTES / TOTAL: 5 MINUTES

It's fall, the leaves are turning, the weather is cooling down, and you are craving pumpkin everything—pumpkin-spiced latte, pumpkin pie, even pumpkin cheesecake. No need to worry about missing these sweet treats when you can have this creamy smoothie, packed with protein and pumpkin flavor and low in sugar. You won't taste the cottage cheese—it will give this smoothie a delectable creamy texture. Pumpkin is packed with nutrients, including the antioxidants vitamin A and beta-carotene and plenty of fiber. Besides adding it to sweet dishes, stir some pumpkin puree into savory dishes like your favorite chili recipe to add a touch of sweetness and thicken the texture.

1 cup low-fat milk or unsweetened soy milk

½ cup pumpkin puree

½ cup low-fat cottage cheese

1 scoop (¼ cup) unflavored or vanilla protein powder

1 teaspoon pumpkin pie spice

1 teaspoon vanilla extract

Post-Op Servings

FL P S G

1 to 3 cups per day

1 In a blender, blend on high speed to combine the milk, pumpkin puree, cottage cheese, protein powder, pumpkin pie spice, and vanilla for 2 to 3 minutes, until the smoothie is smooth and the powder is well dissolved.

2 Pour half the smoothie into a glass and enjoy.

3 Refrigerate any smoothie you don't drink or use right away, and reblend prior to serving. Discard any remaining smoothie after 7 days.

Ingredient tip: *Look for canned pumpkin puree in the baking aisle of your grocery store. Alternatively, make your own from a small pie pumpkin by baking it. Halve the pumpkin; remove and discard the stem, pulp, and seeds; and place the halves cut-side down on a baking sheet coated with the cooking spray. Bake at 350°F for about 60 minutes, until the flesh is tender and can be mashed or pureed.*

Per Serving (1 cup): Calories: 196 Total fat: 2g Sodium: 392mg Total carbs: 17g Sugar: 6g Fiber: 3g Protein: 25g

Sweet Cinnamon-Vanilla Ricotta Cheese

MAKES 2 SERVINGS / PREP: 5 MINUTES / TOTAL: 5 MINUTES

Italian food means comfort, and nothing says comfort food like an Italian dessert. Italian pastries may be out of the question on a weight-loss plan, but this creamy ricotta cheese will have you thinking you just ate velvety, delicious cannoli filling. Sprinkle on a little 100 percent cocoa powder if you'd care for a chocolate twist.

1 cup low-fat
  ricotta cheese

1 teaspoon vanilla extract

1 teaspoon ground
  cinnamon

1 teaspoon
  ground nutmeg

½ teaspoon powdered
  stevia extract

1 In a small container with an airtight lid, use a spoon to mix the ricotta cheese, vanilla, cinnamon, nutmeg, and stevia for 1 minute, until the spices are well distributed among the ricotta cheese.

2 Serve right away or refrigerate overnight for even better flavor.

Post-Op Servings

P ¼ cup

S ½ cup

G ½ to 1 cup

Ingredient tip: *Both ricotta and cottage cheese are excellent sources of protein, and the low-fat versions are low in calories. Plus, they are extremely well tolerated in the first few days and weeks post-op. For a savory ricotta treat, mix some low-sugar spaghetti sauce with the ricotta cheese and have a noodle-less lasagna. Try adding Taco Seasoning (page 174) combined with cottage cheese for a Southwest twist, or stir in some dried onions and chives.*

Per Serving (½ cup): Calories: 116 Total fat: 5g Sodium: 140mg
Total carbs: 6g Sugar: 4g Fiber: 0g Protein: 13g

Pinto Beans and Cheese

MAKES 4 SERVINGS / PREP: 10 MINUTES / COOK: 5 MINUTES / TOTAL: 15 MINUTES

I've counseled many people who craved popular Mexican foods after bariatric surgery. While huge burritos are off limits, the beany, cheesy essence of what makes them so addictive is what you get with this recipe. Vegetarian refried beans are a great source of protein and fiber—two nutrients needed after surgery in high amounts. Beans are a wonderfully inexpensive protein source; keep cans of beans on hand for the early days after surgery or simply to make a meal in a hurry at any time.

1 (15-ounce) can pinto beans, drained and rinsed

1 tablespoon freshly squeezed lime juice

1 teaspoon Taco Seasoning (page 174)

¼ cup shredded cheese, such as Cheddar, Mexican blend, or pepper Jack

Post-Op Servings

Ⓟ ¼ cup

Ⓢ ½ cup

Ⓖ ½ to 1 cup

1　In a small pot over medium-low heat, heat the beans until warm throughout, about 5 minutes. Turn off the heat. Add the lime juice and taco seasoning, and mix to combine.

2　To achieve the desired consistency, use a blender or immersion blender to puree the beans, or mash them with a potato masher.

3　Before serving, top the beans with the cheese and stir to melt.

Post-op tip: *These tasty refried beans are perfect for the puree stage post-op. Add some powdered egg whites or unflavored protein powder to them to increase your protein load for the meal.*

Per Serving (¼ cup): Calories: 123　Total fat: 3g　Sodium: 421mg
Total carbs: 18g　Sugar: 0g　Fiber: 5g　Protein: 7g

Best Scrambled Eggs

MAKES 2 SERVINGS / PREP: 5 MINUTES / COOK: 5 MINUTES / TOTAL: 10 MINUTES

Some of my patients have been fantastic chefs, whereas others haven't known their way around the kitchen. For some, bariatric surgery is a stepping-stone to leaving behind fast food, microwave dinners, and restaurant dining, and an opportunity to learn the very basics about cooking. Here is a recipe to make the perfect scrambled eggs, step by step, and some tips for how to jazz them up.

Nonstick cooking spray

2 eggs

1 tablespoon low-fat milk

½ teaspoon dried thyme

Freshly ground
   black pepper

Post-Op Servings

(P) ¼ cup or 1 egg

(S) ½ cup or 2 eggs

(G) 2 eggs

1 Set a small skillet over medium heat and coat the bottom of the skillet with cooking spray.

2 In a small bowl, beat the eggs lightly with a fork or whisk. Beat in the milk and thyme.

3 Add the egg mixture to the skillet, and turn down the heat to medium-low.

4 Stir the eggs gently and constantly with a rubber spatula for 4 to 5 minutes, until they are fluffy and cooked thoroughly.

5 Season with black pepper and enjoy.

Post-op tip: *After cooking, toss these eggs in the blender to eat on the pureed diet. Eat them immediately while they are still warm. Consider adding additional powdered egg whites (1 tablespoon) to the egg and milk mixture for additional protein. Mix well to dissolve the egg white powder, and you will never know it's there, as the taste does not change. You can add cheese for additional protein as well. When you advance to a soft diet or general consistency diet, add chunks of lean ham or deli turkey to continue to focus on protein. Additional seasonings to jazz up your eggs include rosemary, chives, or dill, or top with salsa or hot sauce.*

Per Serving (¼ cup): Calories: 87 Total fat: 6g Sodium: 83mg
Total carbs: 1g Sugar: 0g Fiber: 0g Protein: 7g

Herbed Chicken Salad with Parsley

MAKES 7 SERVINGS / PREP: 10 MINUTES / TOTAL: 10 MINUTES

Many people find it difficult to include flavorful foods initially after surgery and get bored with eating protein shakes, cottage cheese, and yogurt. Meat is the most protein-dense of all foods, yet initially after surgery many steer away from eating meat because it's extremely filling and dense. Serving meat with a moist sauce can help make it easier to digest. Most chicken salads are laden with high-calorie mayonnaise, but this recipe is packed with herbs, seasonings, and Greek yogurt to give a creamy and tasty finished product.

2 tablespoons low-fat
  plain Greek yogurt

1 tablespoon freshly
  squeezed lemon juice

1 tablespoon dried
  onion flakes

1 teaspoon Dijon mustard

¼ teaspoon dried oregano

¼ teaspoon garlic powder

1½ cups diced cooked
  chicken or 1 (12.5-ounce)
  can chicken breast

Freshly ground black
  pepper

¼ cup chopped fresh
  parsley

1 In a medium bowl, mix together the yogurt, lemon juice, onion flakes, mustard, oregano, and garlic powder until well combined.

2 Add the chicken to the bowl, season with pepper, and mix until everything is well combined and all the chicken is coated. Stir in the parsley.

3 Serve right away or cover and refrigerate overnight to improve the flavors.

Per Serving (¼ cup): Calories: 84 Total fat: 2g Sodium: 43mg
Total carbs: 1g Sugar: 0g Fiber: 0g Protein: 16g

Post-Op Servings

P ¼ cup

S ½ cup

G ½ to 1 cup

Lemon and Dill Tuna Salad

MAKES 3 SERVINGS / PREP: 10 MINUTES / TOTAL: 10 MINUTES

Seafood and fish are nearly always served with lemon. It's a culinary tradition that dates back hundreds of years, as the lemon is essential in neutralizing any fish odor and providing a bright pop of fresh flavor. Fish and seafood are loaded with protein and extremely low in calories—perfect staples for any weight-loss plan. Canned tuna is inexpensive, not to mention extremely convenient and well tolerated after surgery. This tuna salad combines flavorful dill with fresh lemon.

1 (5-ounce) can water-packed tuna

2 tablespoons freshly squeezed lemon juice

1 tablespoon mayonnaise

1 tablespoon plain Greek yogurt

1 teaspoon dried dill

½ teaspoon garlic powder

½ teaspoon Dijon mustard

½ teaspoon freshly ground black pepper

Post-Op Servings

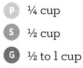

P ¼ cup

S ½ cup

G ½ to 1 cup

1 In a fine-mesh sieve, drain the tuna over the sink. Transfer it to a small bowl.

2 Add the lemon juice, mayonnaise, Greek yogurt, dill, garlic powder, mustard, and pepper to the bowl, and mix with the tuna until well combined.

3 Serve right away or cover and refrigerate overnight to improve the flavors.

Ingredient tip: *There can be many variations to tuna salad to keep it exciting. Here are a few other options to try:*

- *Add pickles, chopped fresh onion, peas, or sunflower seeds on a general diet.*

- *Swap the mayo for avocado to make things extra creamy and get more healthy fat.*

- *Mix plain tuna with one of the seasonings or dressings from chapter 10.*

Per Serving (¼ cup): Calories: 82 Total fat: 4g Sodium: 240mg
Total carbs: 0g Sugar: 0g Fiber: 0g Protein: 11g

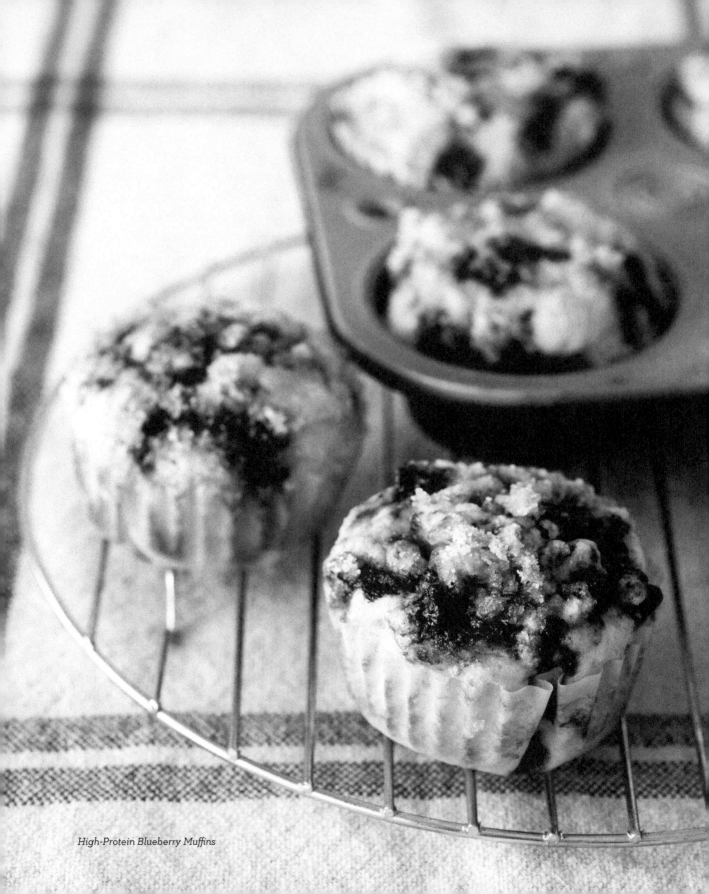

High-Protein Blueberry Muffins

Breakfast

Hearty Slow Cooker Cinnamon Oatmeal

SERVES 10 / PREP: 5 MINUTES / COOK: 7 TO 8 HOURS / TOTAL: 7 TO 8 HOURS

There's a reason oatmeal is a breakfast favorite for so many—it's warming and filling, and it can be totally customized based on the toppings you like. Oats are a hearty grain packed with minerals, fiber, and even some protein. While it's not difficult to cook oats, using a slow cooker is the absolute easiest, most hands-off way to prepare oatmeal. Just put the ingredients in before you go to bed, turn it on, and your oatmeal is ready in the morning. This recipe makes a huge batch so you can easily divide it into small containers to eat throughout the week. It's also easy to freeze and pull out as needed.

8 cups water

2 cups steel-cut oats

1 to 2 teaspoons ground cinnamon

Add-ins for protein (limit to 1 powder to maintain desirable consistency)

½ cup low-fat milk (add before serving or while reheating)

2 tablespoons protein powder, unflavored or vanilla flavored

2 tablespoons nonfat powdered milk or egg white powder

2 tablespoons powdered peanut butter

Add-ins for flavor 8+ weeks post-op (choose 1)

½ cup fresh or frozen berries

½ apple, pear, peach, or banana, peeled and sliced

¼ cup pumpkin puree

2 tablespoons chopped walnuts or almonds

1 In a slow cooker, combine the water, oats, and cinnamon. Cover and cook on low for 7 to 8 hours.

2 Choose and mix in your favorite add-ins before serving.

Ingredient tip: *Oatmeal makes for a great breakfast throughout the year, with your chosen add-ins offering variety so it doesn't get boring. I add apples and pumpkin in the fall, nuts and banana in winter, fresh or frozen berries in spring, and fresh peaches in summer.*

Per serving (¾ cup, no add-ins): Calories: 137 Total fat: 2g Sodium: 0mg Total carbs: 23g Sugar: 0g Fiber: 4g Protein: 6g

Post-Op Servings

P ¼ cup S ½ cup G up to ¾ cup

High-Protein Pancakes

MAKES 4 PANCAKES / PREP: 5 MINUTES / COOK: 5 MINUTES / TOTAL: 10 MINUTES

Pancakes are a weekend breakfast staple, but with the added sugary syrup and butter, they're sure to put you over on your sugar and fat intake for the day. Fortunately, there is a way to prepare this home-style favorite with plenty of protein and retain its desirable cake-like texture. Eat plain, or top with plain yogurt and fresh berries. They are also good topped with unsweetened applesauce.

3 eggs

1 cup low-fat
   cottage cheese

⅓ cup whole-wheat
   pastry flour

1½ tablespoons canola oil

Nonstick cooking spray

Post-Op Servings

S ½ pancake

G 1 to 2 pancakes

1 In large bowl, lightly whisk the eggs.

2 Whisk in the cottage cheese, flour, and canola oil just until combined.

3 Heat a large skillet or griddle over medium heat, and lightly coat with cooking spray.

4 Using a measuring cup, pour ⅓ cup of batter into the skillet for each pancake. Cook for 2 to 3 minutes, or until bubbles appear across the surface of each pancake. Flip the pancakes and cook for 1 to 2 minutes on the other side, until golden brown.

5 Serve immediately.

Per Serving (1 pancake): Calories: 182 Total fat: 10g Sodium: 68mg
Total carbs: 10g Sugar: 1g Fiber: 3g Protein: 12g

Chicken and Cheese Crustless Quiche

MAKES 8 (1-SLICE) SERVINGS
PREP: 15 MINUTES / COOK: 40 MINUTES / TOTAL: 55 MINUTES

Start your day off with a satisfying, protein-packed breakfast like this quiche. Use the leftover grilled chicken from last night's dinner to toss together a fast breakfast. Try adding in chopped vegetables such as bell peppers, onions, and tomatoes to sneak in some extra vegetables. Did I mention that quiche doesn't have to be reserved just for breakfast? Make this for a weeknight meal and keep everyone's palates happy and stomachs full.

Nonstick cooking spray

6 ounces (1¼ cups) grilled, boiled, baked, or canned chicken breast, cubed

4 ounces Swiss cheese, cubed

8 ounces shredded low-fat mozzarella cheese

½ teaspoon dried basil

½ teaspoon dried oregano

¼ teaspoon dried thyme

3 eggs

1 cup low-fat milk

1 Preheat the oven to 400°F.

2 Spray a 9-inch pie pan with cooking spray.

3 Add the chicken and Swiss cheese to the pie pan.

4 Sprinkle the mozzarella over the top, and sprinkle everything with the basil, oregano, and thyme.

5 In a medium bowl, whisk together the eggs and milk. Pour the egg mixture over the chicken and cheese.

6 Bake for 40 minutes, or until lightly browned. Let the quiche rest for 5 minutes, and then serve immediately.

7 The quiche can be refrigerated for up to 1 week. Just reheat the quiche before eating.

Post-Op Servings

Ⓖ 1 slice

Did you know? *Eggs are an excellent source of omega-3 fatty acids. Choose organic cage-free eggs, farm fresh, or omega-3 fortified eggs to get in some of these heart-healthy and anti-inflammatory fats.*

Per Serving (1 slice): Calories: 186 Total fat: 10g Sodium: 360mg
Total carbs: 4g Sugar: 0g Fiber: 0g Protein: 20g

Incredible Deviled Eggs

MAKES 12 DEVILED EGG HALVES
PREP: 10 MINUTES / COOK: 10 MINUTES / TOTAL: 20 MINUTES

It isn't called the incredible, edible egg for nothing! Eggs are inexpensive and packed with protein, vitamins, and minerals, and they are diverse in the kitchen. Deviled eggs don't have to be saved for Easter brunch. They are a great breakfast, midafternoon snack, or add-on to lunch or dinner. Dijon mustard, the secret ingredient in this recipe, jazzes up otherwise plain-tasting eggs. Impress your family with deviled eggs as an appetizer that is quick, easy, and nutritious!

6 eggs

3 tablespoons olive oil mayonnaise

1 tablespoon Dijon mustard

Freshly ground black pepper

Ground paprika, for sprinkling

1 Fill a large pot with water, and bring it to a rapid boil over high heat.

2 Carefully add the eggs to the boiling water using a spoon, and set a timer for 10 minutes.

3 Immediately transfer the eggs from the boiling water to a strainer, and run cold water over the eggs to stop the cooking process.

4 Once the eggs are cool enough to handle, peel them.

5 In a small bowl, mix together the mayonnaise, mustard, and black pepper.

6 Carefully halve each egg lengthwise and scoop out the yolk into the bowl with the mayonnaise mixture. Mix the yolks and mayonnaise mixture together until well combined. The mixture should be smooth and creamy.

7 On a plate or serving platter, carefully place each egg white half cut-side up. Fill each egg half with about 2 teaspoons of filling mixture (divided evenly among the 12 egg halves) and sprinkle each with a little of the paprika.

8 Serve immediately or refrigerate for up to 3 days.

Did you know? *The majority of protein in an egg is contained in the egg white, but the egg yolk contains a small amount of protein, too, as well as the majority of the other nutrients, such as fat-soluble vitamins, minerals, and choline. Choline is an essential nutrient for brain and liver function. You can save on calories by eating just the whites, but eat the entire egg to max out on nutritional value.*

Per Serving (1 deviled egg half) : Calories: 50 Total fat: 4g
Sodium: 90mg Total carbs: 0g Sugar: 0g Fiber: 0g Protein: 3g

Post-Op Servings

 2 deviled egg halves G 4 deviled egg halves

Egg Casserole with Spinach, Peppers, and Tomatoes

SERVES 16 / PREP: 15 MINUTES / COOK: 45 MINUTES / TOTAL: 60 MINUTES

When guests are in from out of town, I hate to spend the entire morning in the kitchen instead of visiting. This egg casserole feeds a crowd, and you can put it together the night before. A lot of people struggle with meeting the recommended servings of fruits and vegetables in a day, especially after surgery when eating such a small amount of food. This is a great way to sneak in some extra veggies first thing in the morning. Not feeding a crowd? No problem. Store the leftovers in small individual containers and refrigerate to reheat for the next few days' breakfasts, and freeze the rest for a later day.

Nonstick cooking spray

2 teaspoons extra-virgin olive oil

1 teaspoon minced garlic

½ red bell pepper, diced

½ yellow bell pepper, diced

4 ounces (1½ cups) diced mushrooms

½ red onion, diced

1 cup spinach

18 eggs

2 tablespoons low-fat milk

½ teaspoon dried oregano

½ teaspoon dried basil

¼ teaspoon red pepper flakes

3 medium tomatoes, diced

1 cup shredded low-fat mozzarella cheese

½ cup shredded Parmesan cheese

1 Preheat the oven to 350°F. Spray a 9-by-13-inch baking dish with cooking spray and set aside.

2 In a large skillet over medium heat, heat the olive oil. When the oil is hot, add the garlic, red and yellow bell peppers, mushrooms, and onion, and sauté for 3 to 5 minutes, until tender.

3 Mix in the spinach, and cook just until it wilts, 1 to 2 minutes. Remove the skillet from the heat.

4 In a large bowl, whisk together the eggs, milk, oregano, basil, and red pepper flakes.

5 Add the cooked vegetables, tomatoes, and mozzarella to the egg mixture. Stir to combine.

6 Pour the mixture into the baking dish and sprinkle the Parmesan cheese over the top.

7 Bake for 35 to 40 minutes, or until lightly browned. Let the casserole rest for 5 minutes before serving.

8 Store leftovers in the refrigerators for up to 1 week. Reheat before eating.

Serving tip: *Customize this egg casserole and keep it interesting by adding other ingredients to vary the filling. Try cooked spicy turkey or chicken sausage. Consider serving it with sliced avocado and Fresh Salsa (page 172) or hot sauce to spice things up even more.*

Per Serving: Calories: 133 Total fat: 8g Sodium: 172mg
Total carbs: 3g Sugar: 1g Fiber: 0g Protein: 11g

Post-Op Servings

G 1 (2-inch by 2-inch) square piece

Mini Egg Muffins with Turkey Bacon

MAKES 24 MINI MUFFINS / PREP: 15 MINUTES / COOK: 25 MINUTES / TOTAL: 40 MINUTES

Love a grab-and-go breakfast but prefer something besides the fast-food drive-through? These mini egg muffins with savory turkey bacon leave you satisfied, but with much less fat and sodium. The best part is that you can make a batch and toss them in the freezer to eat throughout the week or month. Add variations such as spinach, mushrooms, chopped bell peppers, onions, or other favorite omelet ingredients.

Nonstick cooking spray

12 slices cooked turkey bacon, each slice quartered

12 large eggs

¾ cup low-fat milk

½ teaspoon dried oregano

½ teaspoon dried basil

¼ teaspoon freshly ground black pepper

¼ teaspoon garlic powder

1 cup shredded Swiss or Monterey Jack cheese, divided

1 Preheat the oven to 350°F. Spray a 24-cup mini muffin tin with cooking spray.

2 Place 2 turkey bacon pieces in the bottom of each muffin cup.

3 In a large bowl, whisk together the eggs, milk, oregano, basil, pepper, and garlic powder. Mix in ¾ cup of cheese.

4 Fill each muffin cup three-quarters full with the egg mixture. Sprinkle the remaining ¼ cup of cheese on top of the muffins.

5 Bake for 20 to 25 minutes, or until the eggs are set. Let the muffins cool for about 2 minutes before serving.

6 Refrigerate for up to 1 week or freeze for up to 1 month.

Did you know? *Eggs get a bad rap for the high dietary cholesterol content in the yolk. Eating eggs as a part of a balanced diet rich in fiber and low in saturated fat has not been shown to impact blood cholesterol levels. Bottom line: Enjoy your eggs guilt free and limit other foods high in saturated fats to keep a heart-healthy diet.*

Per Serving (2 mini egg muffins) : Calories: 153 Total fat: 8g
Sodium: 232mg Total carbs: 8g Sugar: 1g Fiber: 1g Protein: 13g

Post-Op Servings

Ⓖ 2 mini egg muffins

Overnight Bircher Muesli

SERVES 4 / PREP: 10 MINUTES, PLUS OVERNIGHT TO SOFTEN / TOTAL: OVERNIGHT

Love the comforting and filling quality of hot oatmeal but hate to have any-thing hot during the summer months? Try this recipe for a twist on cold oatmeal. You will be satisfied from your soul to your stomach and start your day feeling refreshed even on the hottest of days. Plus, you don't have to use the stove or microwave. Try it all year-round!

2 cups old-fashioned rolled oats

1 cup low-fat milk

1 cup low-fat plain Greek yogurt

1 tablespoon honey

1 teaspoon ground cinnamon

½ teaspoon vanilla extract

Add-ins for protein (limit to 1 to maintain desirable consistency)

2 tablespoons protein powder, unflavored or vanilla flavored

2 tablespoons nonfat powdered milk or egg white powder

2 tablespoons powdered peanut butter

Other add-ins 8+ weeks post-op (choose 1 or more)

1 cup fresh or frozen berries

1 apple, sliced

2 tablespoons ground flaxseed

2 tablespoons chia seeds

2 tablespoons slivered or chopped almonds

1 In a large container that can be tightly covered, mix together the oats, milk, yogurt, honey, cinnamon, and vanilla. Stir in the add-ins of your choice.

2 Tightly cover and refrigerate the muesli overnight to allow the flavors to meld and the oatmeal to soften.

3 Keep refrigerated and eat within 1 week.

Serving tip: *I love this recipe because you can make it ahead and portion out servings to eat throughout the week. Get some small reusable plastic containers with lids and put individual servings in each container on the first morning. Place in the refrigerator for a quick grab-and-go for your entire family.*

Per Serving (¾ cup) : Calories: 242 Total fat: 4g Sodium: 67mg
Total carbs: 38g Sugar: 9g Fiber: 4g Protein: 13g

Post-Op Servings

P ¼ cup (no add-ins)   **S** ½ cup (no add-ins)   **G** ¾ cup

Smoked Salmon Breakfast Toast

SERVES 4 / PREP: 10 MINUTES / TOTAL: 10 MINUTES

These smoked salmon toasts couldn't be easier to make and are packed with power foods. I recommend skipping the typical bagel and lox, which includes high-fat and low-protein cream cheese, and using avocado instead to load up on heart-healthy fat. The comforting creaminess of the avocado, which is slightly melted on the warm toast, topped with the saltiness of the salmon makes it a winning, healthy combination.

2 tablespoons low-fat plain Greek yogurt

Juice of ½ lemon

1 very ripe avocado

4 slices sprouted-grain bread (100 percent whole-grain)

8 ounces smoked salmon

2 fresh dill sprigs

1 In a small bowl, mix together the yogurt and lemon juice.

2 Cut open the avocado, remove the pit, and scoop out the flesh into the bowl with the yogurt. Mix well. The avocado mixture should be relatively smooth, without any large chunks.

3 Toast the bread.

4 Layer each toast slice with the avocado mixture and 2 ounces of the smoked salmon, and top each with fresh dill. Serve immediately.

Post-Op Servings

G 1 toast

Did you know? *For optimum heart health, the American Heart Association recommends at least 2 servings (4 ounces) per week of fatty fish such as salmon, mackerel, and tuna. Fatty fish contain omega-3 fatty acids, which can help keep cholesterol in check and prevent heart disease and stroke.*

Per Serving (1 toast): Calories: 231 Total fat: 10g Sodium: 646mg Total carbs: 19g Sugar: 2g Fiber: 6g Protein: 18g

High-Protein Blueberry Muffins

MAKES 12 MUFFINS / PREP: 15 MINUTES / COOK: 15 MINUTES / TOTAL: 30 MINUTES

You may be missing your typical fluffy, bakery-fresh blueberry muffins, which melt in your mouth but are loaded with sugar. Here is a healthy muffin that satisfies your taste buds and helps you hit your protein mark. Typical sugary blueberry muffins give you an energy rush and subsequent drop, leaving you craving more. These tasty baked goods will fill you up without the crash and burn from too much sugar.

1½ cups whole-wheat pastry flour

¾ cup unflavored protein powder

2 tablespoons ground flaxseed

1½ teaspoons baking powder

1 teaspoon ground cinnamon

½ teaspoon baking soda

1 cup unsweetened applesauce

½ cup low-fat plain Greek yogurt

2 tablespoons honey

1 teaspoon vanilla extract

1 teaspoon freshly grated lemon zest

3 egg whites

1 cup blueberries, fresh or frozen and thawed

1 Preheat the oven to 350°F. Prepare a 12-cup muffin tin with paper liners and set aside.

2 In a medium bowl, mix together the flour, protein powder, flaxseed, baking powder, cinnamon, and baking soda.

3 In a large bowl, mix together the applesauce, yogurt, honey, vanilla, and lemon zest. Add the egg whites, and gradually stir until just combined.

4 Add the flour mixture to the wet mixture, and stir until just combined. Gently stir in the blueberries.

5 Spoon the batter into the muffin cups, filling them three-quarters full.

6 Bake for 10 to 15 minutes, or until a toothpick inserted into a muffin comes out clean.

7 Place the muffin tin on a wire rack to cool before serving the muffins.

Post-Op Servings

Ⓖ 1 muffin

Ingredient tip: *I love to experiment with muffin and quick bread recipes. I switch around ingredients depending on what I have or what's in season. Try frozen strawberries or cherries. Add ground hemp seed instead of flaxseed. You can even try adding pureed pears (look for baby food) instead of applesauce.*

Per Serving (1 muffin): Calories: 181 Total fat: 1g Sodium: 163mg
Total carbs: 32g Sugar: 8g Fiber: 5g Protein: 12g

Turkey Breakfast Burritos

SERVES 8 / PREP: 10 MINUTES / COOK: 20 MINUTES / TOTAL: 30 MINUTES

The days of grabbing a gas station breakfast burrito on the way to work are long behind you. Yet a savory breakfast sandwich isn't off the table. These breakfast burritos still have fluffy eggs and flavorful sausage, but without all the added sodium and fat. Make these ahead and freeze them, and then toss one in the microwave for a hot breakfast in minutes.

12 eggs

¼ cup low-fat milk

1 pound extra-lean turkey
  breakfast sausage
  (nitrate-free)

Nonstick cooking spray

8 (7- to 8-inch) whole-
  wheat tortillas, such as
  La Tortilla Factory
  low-carb tortillas

Fresh Salsa, for serving
  (page 172)

Optional add-ins

¼ cup sautéed onion, bell
  peppers, spinach, and/
  or mushrooms

¼ cup black beans

2 tablespoons cheese of
  your choice

2 slices chopped
  turkey bacon

1 In a large bowl, whisk together the eggs and milk.

2 In a large skillet over medium-high heat, brown the turkey sausage until cooked thoroughly and no longer pink, about 7 minutes. Transfer the sausage to a bowl and set aside.

3 Use a paper towel to wipe out the skillet, or use a separate large skillet, spray with cooking spray, and set over medium-low heat. Add the egg mixture, and stir gently and constantly with a rubber spatula for 10 to 15 minutes, until the eggs are fluffy and cooked thoroughly.

4 Divide the sausage and scrambled eggs among the tortillas. If you're using any of the add-ins, place them in the tortilla now. Fold over the end of the tortilla, fold in the sides, and roll tightly to close.

5 Serve immediately with the salsa, or place each burrito in a zip-top bag and refrigerate for up to 1 week. To eat, reheat a burrito in the microwave for 60 to 90 seconds. These will also keep well in the freezer for up to 1 month.

Serving tip: *You can make these breakfast burritos a hundred different ways. Switch up the meat, cook different vegetables and mix them in, or try vegetarian proteins like soy crumbles or different beans. By varying the ingredients, you will keep your taste buds interested and keep you away from greasy fast-food burritos that will leave you less than satisfied.*

Per Serving (1 burrito, no add-ins): Calories: 241 Total fat: 10g
Sodium: 743mg Total carbs: 27g Sugar: 1g Fiber: 7g Protein: 20g

Post-Op Servings

S Burrito filling (no tortilla) G ½ to 1 burrito

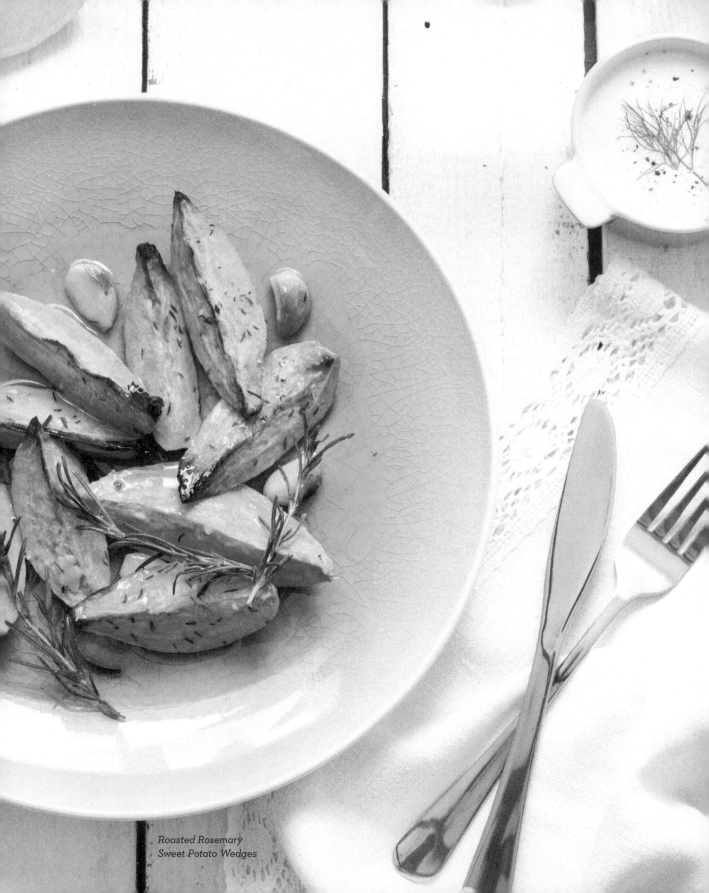

Roasted Rosemary
Sweet Potato Wedges

Vegetables, Dips, and Sides

Roasted Tomatoes, Peppers, and Zucchini with Italian Herbs

MAKES ABOUT 4½ CUPS
PREP: 15 MINUTES / COOK: 25 MINUTES / TOTAL: 40 MINUTES

I know a lot of people who just don't like vegetables. They have tried so many kinds and know the importance of getting them into a balanced diet (high in fiber, low in calories, rich in vitamins, minerals, and antioxidants), but they just can't seem to force them down. When I ask how they usually eat vegetables, the response is often that the vegetables are boiled from a frozen package, or they try to eat them raw, like in a salad. Personally I hardly ever just steam vegetables—I think it gets a tad boring. My favorite way to enjoy vegetables is roasted. Roasting any vegetables in the oven brings out their natural sweet taste and all sorts of other flavors you didn't even know were possible from something so simple. Try these roasted vegetables tonight, and you will instantly become a vegetable lover!

Nonstick cooking spray

1 medium zucchini

2 large tomatoes or 2 cups cherry tomatoes

2 red, green, yellow, or orange bell peppers, or a mix of two

2 tablespoons extra-virgin olive oil

1 teaspoon minced garlic

1 teaspoon dried oregano

1 teaspoon dried basil

½ teaspoon dried thyme

½ teaspoon dried rosemary

1 Preheat the oven to 425°F. Spray a large rimmed baking sheet with cooking spray.

2 To prepare the vegetables, cut off the ends of the zucchini, halve it lengthwise, and then cut lengthwise into thin slices. Remove the ends and cores from the tomatoes, and cut them into 2-inch chunks; if using cherry tomatoes, halve them. Remove the stems from the bell peppers, halve lengthwise, remove the seeds and ribs, and chop into 1-inch chunks.

3 Layer the vegetables on the baking sheet, and sprinkle them with the olive oil, garlic, oregano, basil, thyme, and rosemary. Use a spoon to mix the vegetables and seasonings well.

4 Roast for 20 to 25 minutes, stirring halfway through, until all the vegetables are tender.

5 Serve immediately.

Ingredient tip: *Exchange the vegetables in this recipe for whatever is in season. I love roasting the vegetables in this recipe during the summer months, Brussels sprouts and squash in the fall, broccoli and cauliflower in winter, and asparagus in spring. You can even roast an entire head of cabbage simply by quartering it and sprinkling with olive oil, wrapping very tightly in aluminum foil, and tossing it in the oven for 45 minutes or on the grill.*

Per Serving (½ cup): Calories: 47 Total fat: 3g Sodium: 5mg
Total carbs: 4g Sugar: 2g Fiber: 1g Protein: 1g

Post-Op Servings

 ¼ cup serving   G ½ to 1 cup serving

Roasted Rosemary Sweet Potato Wedges

SERVES 8 / PREP: 15 MINUTES / COOK: 35 MINUTES / TOTAL: 50 MINUTES

French fries are a staple in the typical American diet, and their salty taste is a comfort to many people. After bariatric surgery, greasy fried food is off limits—not only because it's loaded with fat and calories but also because it can make you feel sick. That doesn't mean that you can't enjoy a healthier version of this side dish. These sweet potato wedges are savory and sweet. The longer you bake them, the crunchier they get. So, enjoy your next side of fries—guilt free!

4 medium sweet potatoes
  (about 1½ pounds),
  peeled
6 garlic cloves
2 tablespoons apple
  cider vinegar
2 tablespoons extra-virgin
  olive oil
1 tablespoon chopped
  fresh rosemary
2 to 3 fresh
  rosemary sprigs

Post-Op Servings

G 4 wedges

1 Preheat the oven to 425°F. Line a large rimmed baking sheet with aluminum foil and set aside.

2 Halve each sweet potato lengthwise, and continue slicing each piece lengthwise until you have about 8 wedges per sweet potato.

3 In a large bowl, mix together the garlic cloves, vinegar, olive oil, and chopped rosemary. Add the potato wedges to the bowl, and toss to coat well.

4 Transfer the sweet potatoes and seasonings to the baking sheet, leaving the garlic cloves whole, and place the rosemary sprigs on top of the potato wedges.

5 Roast for 35 minutes, stirring the sweet potatoes every 10 minutes to prevent burning. The potatoes are done when the edges turn crispy and start to brown.

6 Serve immediately.

Per Serving (4 wedges): Calories: 103 Total fat: 3g Sodium: 47mg
Total carbs: 18g Sugar: 4g Fiber: 3g Protein: 1g

Asian Cucumber Salad

MAKES 4½ CUPS / PREP: 15 MINUTES, PLUS 30 MINUTES TO CHILL / TOTAL: 45 MINUTES

Balance out a spicy meal with this cool and refreshing cucumber salad. It serves as a perfect substitute for high-calorie, high-fat creamy coleslaws and salads. This dish will keep for about a week in the refrigerator, so store any leftovers in an airtight container and enjoy this salad throughout the week.

3 medium cucumbers, washed, ends trimmed, and thinly sliced (about 4 cups)

2 scallions, sliced, white and green parts

¼ cup sliced red onion

¼ cup diced red bell pepper

¼ cup rice wine vinegar

2 teaspoons sesame seeds

1 teaspoon honey

½ teaspoon sesame oil

½ teaspoon salt

¼ teaspoon red pepper flakes

1 In a medium bowl, mix together the cucumbers, scallions, red onion, and bell pepper.

2 In a small bowl, whisk together the vinegar, sesame seeds, honey, sesame oil, salt, and red pepper flakes.

3 Pour the dressing over the vegetables, and gently stir until well combined.

4 Cover and chill for at least 30 minutes prior to serving.

Per Serving (½ cup): Calories: 45 Total fat: 1g Sodium: 368mg
Total carbs: 8g Sugar: 5g Fiber: 1g Protein: 1g

Post-Op Servings

G ½ cup serving

Ratatouille over Spaghetti Squash

SERVES 7 / PREP: 15 MINUTES / COOK: 40 MINUTES / TOTAL: 55 MINUTES

You want the pasta, but you don't want all those carbohydrates. You also don't want to leave the meal feeling like an overinflated balloon, since starchy foods tend to make most people feel overly full and uncomfortable after surgery. Spaghetti squash is an excellent alternative to pasta and comes in at a minuscule one-fifth of the calories. Instead of using store-bought spaghetti sauce, which tends to be high in sugar and lacking in diversity of vegetables, try making ratatouille with your bountiful summer vegetables. You can take it a step further by adding cheese, turkey sausage, or baked chicken to get in some protein.

Nonstick cooking spray

1 small (3- to 4-pound) spaghetti squash

¼ cup extra-virgin olive oil

1 teaspoon minced garlic

1 medium yellow onion, diced

1 yellow or orange bell pepper, diced

¼ cup chopped fresh basil

¼ cup chopped fresh parsley

1 teaspoon dried thyme

¼ teaspoon dried rosemary

1 medium eggplant, skin on and cut into ½-inch cubes

1 medium zucchini, cut into ½-inch slices

1 medium yellow squash, cut into ½-inch slices

1½ cups tomatoes, seeded and chopped into ¼-inch dice

1 Preheat the oven to 375°F. Coat a rimmed baking sheet with cooking spray and set aside.

2 Halve the spaghetti squash lengthwise and remove the seeds.

3 Place the squash, cut-side down, on the baking sheet. Roast for about 40 minutes, or until the squash is fork-tender.

4 While the squash is roasting, in a large skillet over medium heat, heat the olive oil. Add the garlic and sauté for about 30 seconds, until fragrant. Add the onion and bell pepper. Sauté the vegetables for about 5 minutes, or until tender. Stir in the basil, parsley, thyme, and rosemary, and mix until well combined.

5 Add the eggplant, zucchini, and yellow squash to the skillet, and sauté for about 10 minutes. Stir in the tomatoes, and cook for an additional 10 minutes, or until all the vegetables are tender. Set aside.

6 Once the roasted squash is cool enough to handle, use a fork to gently scrape out the flesh. The squash should naturally come apart in the shape of spaghetti noodles.

7 Serve the squash noodles with the ratatouille mixture.

Ingredient tip: *If you buy a larger spaghetti squash, you make a bountiful amount of "noodles" to reheat and serve throughout the week with different toppings.*

Per Serving (½ cup): Calories: 136 Total fat: 8g Sodium: 13mg Total carbs: 14g Sugar: 5g Fiber: 6g Protein: 2g

Post-Op Servings

S ¼ cup serving   G ½ to 1 cup serving

Crunchy Roasted Chickpeas

MAKES 4 SERVINGS / PREP: 10 MINUTES / COOK: 20 MINUTES / TOTAL: 30 MINUTES

Many patients struggle to avoid mindless snacking after surgery. Grazing or nibbling on food all day has long been a habit for so many patients I have worked with. Unfortunately, snacking is a way to take in excessive calories, and most foods we snack on—potato chips, pretzels, cookies—are low in nutritional value and high in calories, and we can eat a large portion before our pouch notices we are full. Try to limit snacking as much as possible, but here is a healthy alterative sure to meet your urge to have something crunchy. Roasting these little legumes turns a boring bean into something tasty and flavorful.

Nonstock cooking spray

1 (15.5-ounce) can chickpeas

1 teaspoon extra-virgin olive oil

1 teaspoon garlic powder

1 teaspoon onion powder

½ teaspoon ground cayenne pepper

Post-Op Servings

(G) ⅓ cup

1 Preheat the oven to 400° F. Coat a large rimmed baking sheet with cooking spray and set aside.

2 In a colander or sieve, drain and rinse the chickpeas.

3 In a medium bowl, mix the chickpeas with the olive oil, garlic powder, onion powder, and cayenne pepper.

4 Spread the chickpeas in a single layer on the baking sheet. Roast for 15 to 20 minutes, giving them a stir at least once halfway through the roasting time. The chickpeas are done when they are lightly browned and crispy.

5 Serve immediately.

Serving tip: *Snack on these crunchy chickpeas alone or toss them onto a salad to add flavor, fiber, and protein.*

Per Serving (⅓ cup): Calories: 118 Total fat: 2g Sodium: 330mg Total carbs: 20g Sugar: 0g Fiber: 5g Protein: 5g

Dan's Crock Pickles

MAKES 10 TO 15 SERVINGS

PREP: 15 MINUTES / COOK: 5 MINUTES, PLUS 10 MINUTES TO COOL / TOTAL: 3 TO 5 DAYS

When I work with people who are trying to lose weight, a common complaint is not feeling satisfied after a meal and craving larger quantities of food. One trick is to include foods that satisfy all the taste buds. Pickles have a crisp, sour, delish taste and almost no calories. Here is an easy recipe to make that's better than any jarred pickle. Get fresh pickling cucumbers from the farmers' market or your own garden, if possible. As these crunchy pickles do not contain protein, wait to try them until you advance to the general foods stage of your diet when you are adequately meeting protein needs.

6½ cups water

2 cups distilled
  white vinegar

¼ cup canning salt

4 fresh dill sprigs

3 garlic cloves

10 to 15 pickling
  cucumbers

Post-Op Servings

(G) 1 pickle

1 In a large pot over high heat, bring the water, vinegar, and salt to a boil. When it reaches a rapid boil, turn off the stove and let the liquid sit to cool for 10 minutes.

2 Meanwhile, add the dill sprigs, garlic cloves, and pickling cucumbers to a gallon-size glass jar with an airtight lid.

3 Pour the brine mixture over the cucumbers; they should be completely covered by the liquid. Tightly seal the jar with its lid.

4 Let the pickles stand on the counter for 3 to 5 days. At this point the pickles are ready to eat or be refrigerated. They will keep for 2 months in the refrigerator.

Did you know? *Yogurt isn't the only food with gut-healthy probiotics. Fresh sauerkraut and—you guessed it—pickles are both fermented foods, so they contain healthy bacteria that keep your gastrointestinal tract regular.*

Per Serving (1 pickle): Calories: 9 Total fat: 0g Sodium: 961mg
Total carbs: 2g Sugar: 0g Fiber: 0g Protein: 0g

Mashed Cauliflower

MAKES 3 CUPS / PREP: 10 MINUTES / COOK: 5 MINUTES / TOTAL: 15 MINUTES

Potatoes are a staple starch on many families' plates at dinnertime, but after weight-loss surgery, some people find potatoes make their pouch feel overly full. Not to mention, potatoes are high in carbohydrates and calories compared to most other vegetables. Although potatoes themselves aren't necessarily bad for us, everything we like to put on them—sour cream, butter, bacon bits, cheese—makes the calorie count higher. Try this creamy cauliflower alternative. It's extremely low in both calories and carbohydrates and delivers the same creamy texture as your traditional spuds.

1 large head cauliflower

¼ cup water

⅓ cup low-fat buttermilk (or see step 2 to make homemade buttermilk)

1 tablespoon minced garlic

1 tablespoon extra-virgin olive oil

Post-Op Servings

(P) ¼ cup

(S) (G) ½ cup

1 Break the cauliflower into small florets, and put in a large microwave-safe bowl with the water. Cover and microwave for about 5 minutes, or until the cauliflower is soft. Drain the water from the bowl.

2 You can buy buttermilk in most supermarkets, but it's just as easy to make your own. To make homemade buttermilk, mix 1 teaspoon freshly squeezed lemon juice with ⅓ cup low-fat milk. Let the mixture sit for about 10 minutes, or until the milk begins to thicken.

3 In a blender or food processor, process the buttermilk, cauliflower, garlic, and olive oil on medium speed until the cauliflower is smooth and creamy.

4 Serve immediately.

Ingredient tip: *For even more flavor, microwave the cauliflower with chicken or vegetable broth instead of water and add ½ cup shredded Parmesan cheese when you puree the mixture. You can add protein to this vegetable-based dish by blending in powdered egg whites or unflavored protein powder after the first puree.*

Per Serving (½ cup): Calories: 62 Total fat: 2g Sodium: 54mg
Total carbs: 8g Sugar: 3g Fiber: 3g Protein: 3g

Roasted Red Pepper Hummus

MAKES 14 SERVINGS / PREP: 20 MINUTES / COOK: 5 MINUTES / TOTAL: 25 MINUTES

Most of us love using our condiments to bring flavor to foods—ranch dressing, mayonnaise, catsup, butter. But many of these condiments add excess calories and fat that are not wanted after surgery. Try using hummus as an alternative spread on top of burgers, rolled in lunch meat, or as a dip for raw vegetables. This hummus is so loaded with flavor you can skip the extra sauces and cheese. Not to mention, it includes fresh peppers, which are loaded with immune-building vitamin C.

Nonstick cooking spray

2 red bell peppers, each cut into thirds, stemmed, seeded, and ribs removed

1 (15.5-ounce) can chickpeas, drained and rinsed

Juice of 1 lemon

1 tablespoon minced garlic

3 tablespoons extra-virgin olive oil

2 tablespoons water, plus an additional 1 to 2 tablespoons if needed

½ teaspoon ground cumin

¼ teaspoon dried oregano

¼ teaspoon salt

Post-Op Servings

S G

2 tablespoons

1 Preheat the oven to broil. Coat a large baking sheet with cooking spray and set aside.

2 Place each pepper piece on the baking sheet, inside portion face down. Broil the peppers for about 7 minutes, or until the skin is charred. Remove and set aside to cool.

3 In a food processor or blender, puree the chickpeas, lemon juice, garlic, olive oil, water, cumin, oregano, and salt on high until very smooth, 2 to 3 minutes.

4 When the peppers are cool enough to handle, gently remove the charred portion of the skin and discard. The skin should peel off easily.

5 Cut the roasted peppers into chunks, and add the pieces to the food processor. If you choose, you can set a small portion aside to mince and use as garnish on the finished hummus.

6 Add the peppers to the mixture in the food processor and puree. If needed, add the additional 1 to 2 tablespoons of water to reach your desired consistency.

7 Serve immediately or store in an airtight container for up to 1 week.

Per Serving (2 tablespoons): Calories: 71 Total fat: 3g Sodium: 136mg Total carbs: 9g Sugar: 1g Fiber: 2g Protein: 2g

Mediterranean Layer Dip

MAKES 16 SERVINGS / PREP: 15 MINUTES / TOTAL: 15 MINUTES

This creamy dip packed with flavor will make you feel like you are eating all the toppings from a fresh gyro sandwich. Bring this to your next work potluck to impress your colleagues with a healthy and flavorful dip that is much lower in calories and higher in nutrients than the typical spreads. You can even save the leftovers and use as a topping to jazz up a plain chicken breast.

10 ounces plain or garlic hummus or Roasted Red Pepper Hummus (page 73)

1 tomato, diced

½ cup diced cucumber

½ cup low-fat plain Greek yogurt

½ lemon, seeded

¼ teaspoon ground paprika

1 (14.5-ounce) can water-packed artichoke hearts, drained, rinsed, and chopped into ¼-inch pieces

½ medium red onion, chopped

¼ cup feta cheese crumbles

1 cup pitted Kalamata olives, finely chopped

2 tablespoons chopped fresh parsley

1 In an 8-by-8-inch square dish, spread the hummus evenly along the bottom. Layer the tomato and cucumber over the hummus.

2 Spoon the yogurt over the vegetables and spread it evenly using a rubber spatula. Squeeze the juice of the lemon over the yogurt. Sprinkle with the paprika.

3 Layer the chopped artichokes, red onion, and feta cheese over the yogurt. Top with the olives and parsley.

4 Serve this dip with fresh vegetables, whole-grain crackers, or whole-grain pita chips.

Per Serving (¼ cup): Calories: 93 Total fat: 5g Sodium: 381mg
Total carbs: 8g Sugar: 0g Fiber: 2g Protein: 4g

Post-Op Servings

(G) ¼ cup

Spinach and Artichoke Dip

MAKES 16 SERVINGS
PREP: 10 MINUTES / COOK: ABOUT 10 MINUTES / TOTAL: 20 MINUTES

Need an appetizer for your next football party or holiday gathering? Look no further than this spinach-artichoke dip. It has the same creamy, cheesy texture as the favorite dip at your local bar or eatery, but without the extra fat and calories. Don't be fearful of the secret ingredient—tofu. You and your guests will have no clue it's mixed inside. It's crucial for adding protein, keeping the calorie count per serving down, and giving this dip its ultracreamy texture. This recipe came to me by way of fellow registered dietitian Joelle Lefevre, and I haven't stopped recommending it since!

1 (14.5-ounce) can water-packed artichoke hearts, drained

8 ounces shredded low-fat mozzarella cheese

8 ounces shredded Parmesan cheese

1 tablespoon hot sauce

8 ounces silken tofu

2 cups fresh spinach (about 2 handfuls)

16 ounces low-fat plain Greek yogurt

2 teaspoons minced garlic

1 teaspoon seasoning salt

Post-Op Servings

(G) ¼ cup

1 Chop the artichokes into small pieces. Try using clean kitchen scissors to easily cut them into small pieces.

2 In a large bowl, use a hand mixer on low speed to mix the artichokes, mozzarella cheese, Parmesan cheese, hot sauce, tofu, spinach, yogurt, garlic, and salt until well combined, 2 to 3 minutes.

3 Before serving, heat the dip on the stove, in the microwave, or in a mini slow cooker until the cheese melts and the spinach is wilted. The time will vary depending on how you heat the dip.

4 Serve with raw vegetables or whole-grain crackers.

Serving tip: *This dip makes a huge batch—enough to feed a crowd. Save the leftovers and spoon over raw chicken breasts prior to baking them in the oven, making a tasty spinach-artichoke chicken dinner.*

Per Serving (¼ cup): Calories: 139 Total fat: 7g Sodium: 551mg
Total carbs: 6g Sugar: 2g Fiber: 1g Protein: 13g

Greek Ranch Dip

MAKES 2 CUPS
PREP: 10 MINUTES, PLUS AT LEAST 30 MINUTES TO CHILL / TOTAL: 40 MINUTES

This creamy ranch dip will jazz up your favorite raw vegetables or salad. Grilled or baked chicken breasts make great dippers, too—the dip adds wonderful flavor and keeps the chicken moist. Try mixing the dip with a can of tuna for a twist on your traditional tuna salad. No matter how closely you watch protein intake while keeping fat and sugar consumption low, you can't escape the fact that veggies and healthy meats are important to your post-op diet. This easy dip is a delicious and semi-indulgent way of making sure we eat nature's healthiest foods, which may not be the most flavorful on their own.

2 tablespoons Ranch
Seasoning (page 173)
16 ounces low-fat plain
Greek yogurt

In a small bowl, mix the ranch seasoning with the yogurt. Cover and refrigerate overnight or for at least 30 minutes prior to serving to bring out the full flavor of the dip.

Post-Op Servings

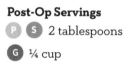 2 tablespoons

G ¼ cup

Ingredient tip: *If you're making this dip during your puree stage, add in some tuna or chicken before blending to add both protein and flavor.*

Per Serving (¼ cup): Calories: 25 Total fat: 1g Sodium: 14 mg
Total carbs: 0g Sugar: 0g Fiber: 0g Protein: 3g

Slow Cooker Boston Baked Beans

SERVES 7 / PREP: 10 MINUTES, PLUS OVERNIGHT TO SOAK / COOK: 7 TO 8 HOURS / TOTAL: OVERNIGHT, PLUS 7 TO 8 HOURS, 30 MINUTES

Many people love baked beans as a side dish but the traditional versions are loaded with sugar and greasy fat from bacon. This recipe is healthier and is tastier than any canned version you will find at the grocery store. It requires a day of preplanning since you need to soak the beans overnight—but it takes about only 10 minutes to throw together since you probably have most of these basic ingredients in your pantry already.

½ pound dried
  pinto beans

1 (15-ounce) can
  tomato sauce

1¾ cups water

2½ tablespoons low-
  sodium soy sauce or
  Bragg Liquid Aminos

2 tablespoons apple
  cider vinegar

1 tablespoon molasses

1 tablespoon
  ground cumin

2 teaspoons minced garlic

1½ teaspoons Chili
  Powder (page 175)

½ teaspoon onion powder

¼ teaspoon dried
  mustard powder

¼ teaspoon salt

1 In a medium bowl, cover the beans by at least 2 inches with enough cold water. Cover, refrigerate, and soak overnight.

2 Drain and rinse the beans in a colander or sieve.

3 In the slow cooker, combine the beans, tomato sauce, water, soy sauce, vinegar, molasses, cumin, garlic, chili powder, onion powder, mustard powder, and salt. Cover the slow cooker, and cook the beans on low for 7 to 8 hours. The beans are done when the sauce is thick and the beans are tender.

4 Turn the slow cooker temperature to warm and let the baked beans sit for 30 minutes prior to serving.

Did you know? *Beans are an excellent source of soluble fiber. Soluble fiber is important for heart health since it helps transport cholesterol out of the body. Include a serving of beans or legumes in your diet several times per week to help control blood cholesterol levels.*

Per Serving (½ cup): Calories: 136 Total fat: 0g Sodium: 606mg
Total carbs: 26g Sugar: 5g Fiber: 6g Protein: 8g

Post-Op Servings

P ¼ cup

S G ½ cup

Mixed Vegetable Stir-Fry with Sesame Tofu

CHAPTER FIVE

Vegetarian Dinners

Corn, Edamame, and Quinoa Salad

SERVES 10 / PREP: 15 MINUTES / COOK: 10 MINUTES / TOTAL: 25 MINUTES

Beans and legumes are excellent sources of vegetarian protein, but so many patients find them boring to eat because they don't know how to prepare them in a way that tastes good. This recipe is packed with a one-two protein punch from the beans and quinoa and topped with a scrumptious dressing, including refreshing flavors from cilantro and lemon. Use this as a side dish or serve as a meal all on its own. You will never miss the meat.

⅔ cup water

⅓ cup quinoa

3 cups fresh corn (about 3 cobs)

1 (14.5-ounce) can black beans, drained and rinsed

1 (15.5-ounce) can chickpeas, drained and rinsed

2 cups frozen shelled edamame, thawed

1 medium red bell pepper, cut into ¼-inch slices

¼ cup reduced-sodium soy sauce or Bragg Liquid Aminos

3 tablespoons freshly squeezed lemon juice

3 tablespoons rice vinegar

2 tablespoons Dijon mustard

2 tablespoons extra-virgin olive oil

½ cup chopped fresh cilantro

4 teaspoons minced garlic

6 scallions, finely sliced

1 In a small saucepan, heat the water and quinoa over high heat. When the water comes to a boil, cover, reduce the heat to low, and cook the quinoa for 10 to 12 minutes, or until the quinoa is tender and the water is absorbed. Remove the pan from the heat, fluff the quinoa with a fork, and set aside.

2 In a medium serving bowl, mix together the corn, black beans, chickpeas, edamame, and red bell pepper.

3 In a small bowl, whisk together the soy sauce, lemon juice, rice vinegar, mustard, olive oil, cilantro, garlic, and scallions.

4 Stir the quinoa into the corn and bean mixture, drizzle with the dressing, and mix well.

5 For the best flavor, refrigerate the salad for at least 30 minutes before serving to let the flavors blend together.

Did you know? *Soybeans (edamame) are one of the few vegetarian sources of 100 percent complete, containing all essential amino acids—important for maintaining muscle mass. Soy has also been shown to help with lowering cholesterol, and soy products contain cancer-protective isoflavones. Toss edamame into your next salad or stir-fry, or try soy milk or soy nuts.*

Per Serving (1 cup): Calories: 229 Total fat: 5g Sodium: 757mg Total carbs: 36g Sugar: 6g Fiber: 8g Protein: 10g

Post-Op Servings

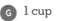 1 cup

Naked Burrito Salad

SERVES 6 / PREP: 10 MINUTES / COOK: 10 MINUTES / TOTAL: 20 MINUTES

Burritos do not have to be off limits when you put a simple twist on them to reduce carbohydrates and fat. Most burritos at fast-food restaurants come with tortillas nearly as big as your head. For weight loss we have to do without all those extra carbohydrates and calories—but you won't even miss them when you taste this salad's seasonings of cumin and oregano with black beans and corn. This is a great salad to take for lunch and use up leftover toppings from the previous night's taco feast.

Nonstick cooking spray

½ cup soy crumbles, GMO-free, such as Beyond Meat or Gardein brands

3 tablespoons water, plus 1 to 2 tablespoons additional if needed

1 teaspoon Taco Seasoning (page 174)

½ cup canned black beans, drained and rinsed

½ cup corn kernels, fresh off the cob or thawed frozen

3 cups chopped romaine lettuce

¾ cup diced tomatoes

½ red bell pepper, diced

½ cup diced red onion

¼ cup Avocado-Lime Dressing (page 166)

1 Spray a small skillet with cooking spray and place it over medium heat. Add the soy crumbles, water, and taco seasoning. Stir constantly until some of the water is absorbed.

2 Add the black beans and corn to the skillet, and cook until the soy crumbles are heated thoroughly and all the water is absorbed, 5 to 7 minutes. Note: You may need to add 1 to 2 tablespoons more water to reach your desired texture; the soy crumbles should be soft but moist, similar in appearance to cooked ground beef. Remove the skillet from the heat and set aside

3 Divide the lettuce, tomatoes, bell pepper, and onion evenly among your serving plates. Top each with an equal amount of the soy crumbles, bean, and corn mixture. Drizzle each with the dressing and serve immediately.

Serving tip: *Pack this for lunch the night before so you'll have no excuse to skip a balanced meal. Keep the salad ingredients, soy crumble-bean-corn mixture, and dressing in separate airtight containers, and grab the containers from the refrigerator as you head out to work.*

Per Serving (1 cup): Calories: 167 Total fat: 3g Sodium: 336mg
Total carbs: 27g Sugar: 2g Fiber: 8g Protein: 8g

Post-Op Servings
G 1 to 2 cups

Sweet Potato and Black Bean Soup

SERVES 10 / PREP: 15 MINUTES / COOK: 35 MINUTES / TOTAL: 50 MINUTES

Sweet potatoes are more than a side dish at Thanksgiving; they are great cooked into this bean soup. Mix up a pot of this soup and serve it topped with fresh chopped cilantro and low-fat plain Greek yogurt. Your taste buds will be delighted with the slightly spicy Southwest flavor, and your gut will appreciate the extra fiber from the black beans, which are a great alternative to meat sources of protein. I am normally not a huge fan of recommending soups after surgery, since they tend to be mostly liquid, low in protein, and unable to keep you full for very long; however, this soup is hearty and thick and will keep you full and satisfied for hours.

1 tablespoon extra-virgin olive oil

1 red bell pepper, diced

1 green bell pepper, diced

½ jalapeño pepper, diced

1 medium yellow or white onion, diced

2 teaspoons minced garlic

2 teaspoons Chili Powder (page 175)

1 teaspoon ground cumin

½ teaspoon dried oregano

½ teaspoon ground paprika

2 medium sweet potatoes, peeled and cut into ½-inch cubes (about 4 cups)

2 (14.5-ounce) cans black beans, drained and rinsed

1 (28-ounce) can diced tomatoes or 2½ cups chopped fresh tomatoes

½ cup corn kernels, fresh or frozen

1½ cups vegetable broth

Low-fat plain Greek yogurt, for garnish (optional)

¼ cup chopped fresh cilantro, for garnish (optional)

1 In a large stockpot over medium heat, heat the olive oil. Add the red and green bell peppers, jalapeño, onion, and garlic. Sauté until tender, 3 to 5 minutes.

2 Add the chili powder, cumin, oregano, and paprika, and stir until the vegetables are well coated.

3 Add the sweet potatoes, beans, tomatoes, corn, and broth.

4 Bring the soup to a boil, and then reduce the heat to a simmer. Cover and simmer the soup for 30 minutes.

5 Remove the pot from the heat. Garnish each bowl of soup with the Greek yogurt (if using) for added protein and the cilantro (if using) for a flavor boost, and serve.

Ingredient tip: *Looking for an even bigger protein boost? Add 1 cup of cooked chicken breast, mix well into the soup, and cook for the last 10 minutes to make sure it's heated thoroughly. As with other soups, if you're enjoying this during the puree stage, boost protein by adding 1 to 2 tablespoons of egg white powder or unflavored protein powder after the soup has cooled but before adding it to the blender.*

Per Serving (1 cup): Calories: 140 Total fat: 2g Sodium: 433mg Total carbs: 24g Sugar: 5g Fiber: 9g Protein: 8g

Post-Op Servings

P ¼ cup   S ½ cup   G 1 to 2 cups

Garden Vegetable Cheezy Chili

SERVES 12 / PREP: 15 MINUTES / COOK: 30 MINUTES / TOTAL: 45 MINUTES

Chili is an easy go-to meal for many families. It doesn't have to be packed with high-fat ground beef and sour cream to be good. Grab these fresh ingredients from your local farmers' market, and in just a few steps you'll have a simple but delicious chili that even the most inexperienced cook can make. This chili is as appealing to the eyes as to the stomach with tons of tasty vegetables and flavorful seasonings. This meal is great to feed a crowd or freeze for a future date and reheat.

2 teaspoons extra-virgin olive oil

2 teaspoons minced garlic

1 large green bell pepper, diced

2 cups sliced mushrooms

1 cup chopped onion

1 (14.5-ounce) can diced tomatoes or 2 cups diced fresh tomatoes

1 (8-ounce) can tomato sauce

2 tablespoons Chili Powder (page 175)

1 medium zucchini, thinly sliced

1 medium yellow summer squash, thinly sliced

2 (15-ounce) cans red kidney beans, drained and rinsed

1 (10-ounce) package frozen corn or 1¾ cups fresh corn kernels

1 cup shredded Cheddar cheese (optional)

½ cup low-fat plain Greek yogurt (optional)

1   In a large skillet or stockpot over medium heat, heat the olive oil.

2   Add the garlic, green bell pepper, mushrooms, and onion, and sauté until tender, about 5 minutes.

3   Stir in the diced tomatoes, tomato sauce, and chili powder. Bring the liquid to a boil, and then reduce the heat to low. Stir in the zucchini, yellow squash, kidney beans, and corn. Cover and simmer for 15 to 20 minutes.

4   Remove the skillet from the heat. Garnish each bowl with some Cheddar cheese (if using) and Greek yogurt (if using) and serve.

Ingredient tip: *Boost protein during the early post-op puree stage by adding 1 to 2 tablespoons of egg white powder or unflavored protein powder before blending.*

Per Serving (1 cup): Calories: 199 Total fat: 3g Sodium: 418mg
Total carbs: 35g Sugar: 5g Fiber: 8g Protein: 8g

Post-Op Servings

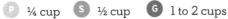

ⓟ ¼ cup   Ⓢ ½ cup   Ⓖ 1 to 2 cups

Vegetable Lentil Soup

SERVES 8 / PREP: 10 MINUTES / COOK: 45 MINUTES / TOTAL: 55 MINUTES

With only a few basic ingredients, this vegetarian delight is easy to whip up. The recipe makes a large batch, which is perfect for several meals and for freezing leftovers. This soup is packed with fiber-rich lentils and vegetables to keep you fueled up, full, and energized. The cumin and coriander seasonings give the lentils a warm flavor to keep you toasty on a cold winter day.

2 tablespoons extra-virgin olive oil

1 cup onion, chopped

½ cup carrots, cut into ½-inch chunks

½ cup celery, cut into ¼-inch chunks

1 teaspoon minced garlic

1 pound dried lentils rinsed

½ teaspoon ground coriander

½ teaspoon ground cumin

¼ teaspoon red pepper flakes

1 cup chopped tomatoes

4 cups vegetable broth

4 cups water

Low-fat plain Greek yogurt, for garnish (optional)

1 In a large stockpot over medium heat, heat the olive oil. Add the onion, carrots, celery, and garlic, and sauté until tender, 5 to 7 minutes.

2 Add the lentils, coriander, cumin, and red pepper flakes. Mix well and stir for 1 to 2 minutes, until all ingredients are coated well with the seasonings.

3 Add the tomatoes, broth, and water to the pot. Bring to a simmer, then cover the pot and cook the soup for 35 to 40 minutes.

4 Remove the pot from the heat. Use an immersion blender to puree the soup to your desired consistency. Alternatively, let the soup cool for 10 minutes, then puree it in batches in a blender.

5 Garnish each bowl of soup with a dollop of Greek yogurt (if using) and serve.

Ingredient tip: *If you're cooking during the post-op puree stage, add 1 to 2 tablespoons of egg white powder or unflavored protein powder after cooking to increase the protein content.*

Per Serving (1 cup): Calories: 252 Total fat: 4g Sodium: 281mg Total carbs: 39g Sugar: 4g Fiber: 19g Protein: 15g

Post-Op Servings

P ¼ cup

S ½ cup

G 1 to 2 cups

Vegetable Tortilla Pizza for One

SERVES 1 / PREP: 15 MINUTES / COOK: 10 MINUTES / TOTAL: 25 MINUTES

Who doesn't love pizza? It's a convenient and quick meal that tastes delicious. Just because you had bariatric surgery does not mean you can never have pizza again—just maybe not the Chicago deep-dish version. Pizza can still be delicious without extra-greasy meat and a thick, doughy crust. Try this recipe for a simple pizza for one. The tortilla crust turns out extra crispy in the hot oven, and the seasonings give the vegetables lots of Italian flavor.

1 (7- to 8-inch) whole-wheat tortilla, such as La Tortilla Factory low-carb tortillas

1 teaspoon extra-virgin olive oil

¼ teaspoon dried oregano

¼ teaspoon dried rosemary

¼ teaspoon garlic powder or minced fresh garlic

¾ cup Roasted Tomatoes, Peppers, and Zucchini with Italian Herbs (page 64)

¼ cup shredded Parmesan cheese

¼ cup shredded low-fat mozzarella cheese

1 small handful arugula

Post-Op Servings

G 1 tortilla pizza

1 Preheat the oven to 400°F.

2 Brush the tortilla lightly with the olive oil using a pastry or marinade brush. Sprinkle the oregano, rosemary, and garlic over the tortilla, and then layer the roasted vegetables across the tortilla.

3 Cover the vegetables with the Parmesan and mozzarella cheeses, and top the pizza with the arugula.

4 Carefully transfer the pizza directly onto the oven rack, and bake it for 10 minutes, or until the cheese melts, the tortilla edges are crisp, and the arugula is wilted.

5 Carefully remove the pizza from the oven, cut it into fourths for easy handling, and enjoy.

Ingredient tip: *Make variations with different vegetables and seasonings. Try a Mexican pizza by spreading Pinto Beans and Cheese (page 40) on the tortilla and topping it with Taco Seasoning (page 174), cooked ground turkey, sautéed peppers and onions, and Cheddar cheese. If you are looking for something more traditional, add tomato sauce to the crust, then top with seasonings, cooked Italian turkey sausage, mushrooms, and onions.*

Per Serving: Calories: 275 Total fat: 15g Sodium: 725mg
Total carbs: 13g Sugar: 0g Fiber: 8g Protein: 22g

Cauliflower "Mac" and Cheese

SERVES 8 / PREP: 10 MINUTES / COOK: 45 MINUTES / TOTAL: 55 MINUTES

Mac and cheese is a staple for kids and adults alike. For many, it's the ultimate comfort food. With all that high-fat cheese sauce and high-carb pasta, traditional versions are out of the question after bariatric surgery, but this recipe serves up a fantastic meal that's sure to please kids of all ages. Enjoy this tasty dish as a side or the main event. Cauliflower has the look and feel of pasta but with virtually no carbs. This can easily be made ahead of time to enjoy at a later date, and it freezes well.

1 head cauliflower, broken into florets

1 cup low-fat cottage cheese

1 cup low-fat plain Greek yogurt

1 egg

½ teaspoon turmeric powder

½ teaspoon Dijon mustard

¼ teaspoon garlic powder

2 ounces (½ cup) shredded aged white Cheddar cheese

2 ounces (½ cup) shredded Cheddar cheese

1 Preheat the oven to 350°F.

2 Fill a medium pot one-third full with water, and place a steamer basket inside. Bring the water to a boil over high heat.

3 Add the cauliflower to the steamer basket, cover the pot, and reduce the heat to a gentle boil. Steam the cauliflower for 10 to 15 minutes, or until the florets are soft. Alternatively, you can steam the cauliflower in the microwave for about 7 minutes.

4 While the cauliflower steams, in a medium bowl, mix together the cottage cheese, yogurt, egg, turmeric, mustard, and garlic powder.

5 Drain the cauliflower in a large colander, and gently mash it with a potato masher to drain out excess water.

6 Stir the cauliflower pieces into the cottage cheese mixture. Add the Cheddar cheeses and mix well.

7 Transfer the cauliflower mixture to an 8-by-8-inch or 11-by-7-inch baking dish. Bake for about 30 minutes. The cauliflower "mac" and cheese is finished when the edges begin to brown.

8 Serve immediately.

Ingredient tip: *Instead of your traditional Cheddar cheese, try something with a bit more flavor—Gruyère, aged Cheddar, smoked Gouda, or Havarti. By using a more flavorful cheese, you may find yourself satisfied with a smaller portion of the finished recipe.*

Per Serving (½ cup): Calories: 147 Total fat: 7g Sodium: 263mg
Total carbs: 8g Sugar: 4g Fiber: 2g Protein: 13g

Post-Op Servings

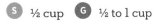 ½ cup ½ to 1 cup

Vegetarian Tacos with Lentils

SERVES 12 / PREP: 15 MINUTES / COOK: 40 MINUTES / TOTAL: 55 MINUTES

These tacos are one of my all-time favorites. The lentils for the filling are delicious in a taco shell or can be used to top a salad or be eaten by themselves. The seasonings and salsa give this meal a ton of great flavor. The texture even resembles ground beef, so the carnivores in the house won't miss the meat. I love this meal because it's inexpensive to make and produces a big batch, which is easy to reheat as leftovers or freeze for another night when you just don't want to cook.

1 teaspoon extra-virgin olive oil

1 cup chopped onion

1 teaspoon minced garlic

1 cup dried lentils, rinsed

1 tablespoon Chili Powder (page 175)

2 teaspoons ground cumin

1 teaspoon dried oregano

2½ cups vegetable broth

1 cup Fresh Salsa (page 172)

12 (7- to 8-inch) whole-grain taco shells, such as La Tortilla Factory low-carb taco shells

1½ cups finely shredded romaine lettuce

1½ cups shredded Cheddar cheese

¼ cup low-fat plain Greek yogurt

1 In a large skillet over medium heat, heat the olive oil. Add the onion and garlic, and sauté until tender, 2 to 3 minutes.

2 Add the lentils, chili powder, cumin, and oregano, and cook for 1 minute, stirring to coat the lentils well.

3 Add the broth and bring to a boil. Reduce the heat to a simmer, cover, and simmer for 25 to 30 minutes.

4 Uncover the skillet and continue to cook for 6 to 8 minutes more to thicken the mixture.

5 Mash the lentils lightly using a potato masher. Stir in the salsa until well combined.

6 To serve, spoon ¼ cup of filling into each tortilla shell. Top each with the lettuce, cheese, and 1 teaspoon of yogurt.

Per Serving (1 taco): Calories: 175 Total fat: 7g Sodium: 592mg Total carbs: 17g Sugar: 2g Fiber: 9g Protein: 11g

Post-Op Servings

P ¼ cup (filling only, no toppings or shell)

S ½ cup (filling only)

G 1 taco

Butternut Squash Casserole with Mozzarella Cheese

SERVES 8 / PREP: 15 MINUTES / COOK: 45 MINUTES / TOTAL: 1 HOUR

Most butternut squash casseroles are topped with sugary marshmallows or coated with brown sugar and butter, but you don't have to sacrifice this comfort dish completely. Butternut squash has a sweet, savory flavor when baked all on its own. Skip the sugar, add some basil, garlic, and mozzarella cheese, and you have a new, even more delicious version. Serve it at your Thanksgiving table or just to make a regular Monday dinner special.

Nonstick cooking spray

1 tablespoon extra-virgin olive oil

1 large onion, chopped

2 tablespoons minced garlic

1 medium (2- to 3-pound) butternut squash, peeled, seeds and pulp removed, and chopped into 1-inch cubes

3 eggs

¾ cup low-fat plain Greek yogurt

⅓ cup chopped fresh basil

¼ teaspoon freshly ground black pepper

2 cups shredded low-fat mozzarella cheese, divided

1 Preheat the oven to 425°F. Coat a 9-by-13-inch casserole dish with cooking spray and set aside.

2 In a large skillet over medium heat, heat the olive oil. Add the onion and garlic, and sauté until the onion is soft, about 7 minutes.

3 Add the squash and cook for about 10 minutes, or until tender.

4 Transfer the squash and onion to the casserole dish.

5 In a small bowl, lightly whisk the eggs. Whisk in the yogurt, basil, pepper, and 1 cup of mozzarella cheese.

6 Pour the egg mixture over the squash, and top the casserole with the remaining 1 cup of mozzarella cheese.

7 Bake for 30 minutes, or until the squash is very tender and the cheese begins to bubble and lightly brown.

8 Serve immediately.

Post-Op Servings

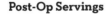

(S) ½ cup

(G) ½ to 1 cup

Per Serving (½ cup): Calories: 192 Total fat: 8g Sodium: 190mg
Total carbs: 20g Sugar: 5g Fiber: 3g Protein: 12g

Mixed Vegetable Stir-Fry with Sesame Tofu

SERVES 6
PREP: 15 MINUTES, PLUS 30 MINUTES TO DRAIN / COOK: 25 MINUTES
TOTAL: 1 HOUR, 10 MINUTES

Many patients ask me for tips on getting more vegetables into their diets. It can be difficult post-op because most people tend to tolerate cooked vegetables better than raw vegetables, at least initially. Yet steamed vegetables get boring and bland after a while. Enter this delicious, flavorful stir-fry. And tofu is a great substitute for meat—it's heart healthy, loaded with protein, and inexpensive, and it soaks up the flavor of all the seasonings it's cooked in. When you use the extra-firm variety and sauté it, it even has the same texture as meat!

1 (14-ounce) package extra-firm tofu

3 teaspoons sesame oil, divided

1 tablespoon sesame seeds, plus additional for garnish

1 medium bok choy, stems chopped into ½-inch pieces, leaves diced

½ large red bell pepper, seeded and chopped

1 red banana pepper

1 cup chopped broccoli florets

1 cup sugar snap peas

1 cup Quick Stir-Fry Sauce (page 168)

¼ cup chopped fresh cilantro, for garnish

1 Drain the tofu and place it in a paper towel–lined plate or bowl. Cover with several layers of paper towel or a clean dish towel, and set a can on top for added weight. Let the tofu sit for 30 minutes to drain some of its excess water.

2 Place the tofu on a clean cutting board. Halve lengthwise and cut into 1-by-2-inch cubes.

3 In a large nonstick pan over medium heat, heat 1½ teaspoons of sesame oil.

4 When the oil is very hot, add the tofu cubes and cook until lightly browned on all sides, 10 to 15 minutes. During the last 2 minutes, add the sesame seeds and stir frequently to prevent them from burning. Transfer the tofu and sesame seeds to a bowl and set aside.

5   In the same pan over medium heat, add the remaining 1½ teaspoons of sesame oil. Once the oil is very hot, add the bok choy, red bell pepper, banana pepper, broccoli, and snap peas. Cook, stirring frequently, for 10 minutes, until the vegetables are crisp-tender.

6   Add the stir-fry sauce and tofu to the pan, and stir to coat the tofu and vegetables.

7   Serve the stir-fry garnished with the cilantro and a sprinkle of sesame seeds.

Serving tip: *Try this stir-fry without serving it over rice or noodles to keep it low carb. If you tolerate rice without issues, try limiting the rice to only a ¼-cup serving, and make sure to choose brown rice.*

Per Serving (1 cup): Calories: 181 Total fat: 9g Sodium: 659mg
Total carbs: 13g Sugar: 6g Fiber: 6g Protein: 12g

Post-Op Servings

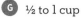 ½ to 1 cup

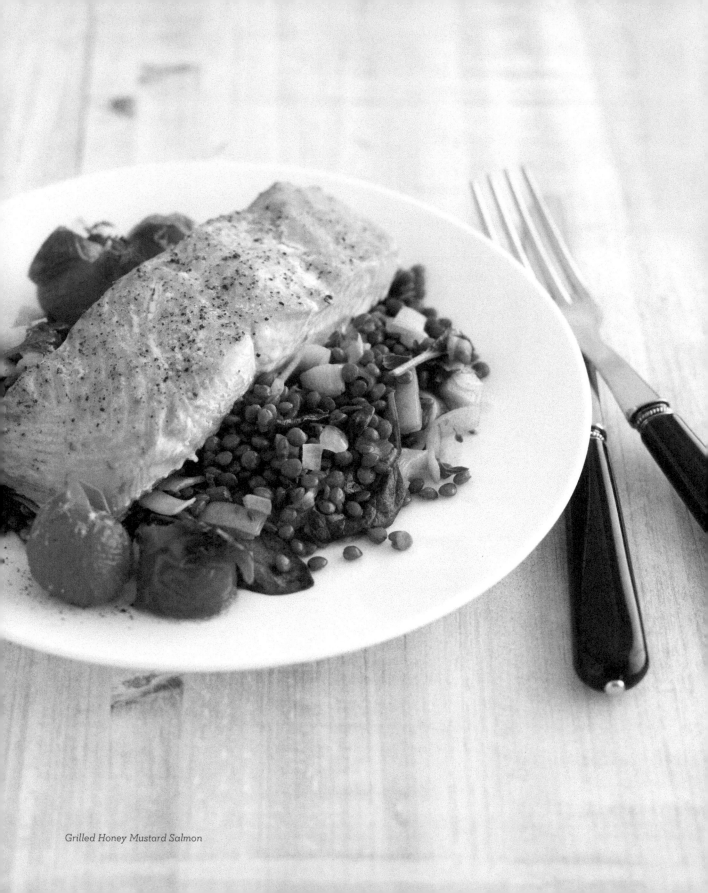

Grilled Honey Mustard Salmon

Fish and Seafood Dinners

Szechuan Shrimp Zoodle Bowl

SERVES 6 / PREP: 15 MINUTES / COOK: 15 MINUTES / TOTAL: 30 MINUTES

Keeping your carb intake low post-op is key, so that means no pasta. But noodle bowls are all the rage, and this recipe lets you enjoy the taste without the high-starch ramen noodles. Try this version made with zoodles (zucchini noodles) and shrimp. It's packed with protein, vegetables, and lots of flavorful spices. Not to mention shrimp is one of the lowest-calorie protein sources you can find.

1 pound zucchini (about
   3 medium zucchini)
2 teaspoons extra-virgin
   olive oil
¼ cup water
2 tablespoons catsup
   (choose a version
   without high-fructose
   corn syrup)
1 tablespoon soy sauce
2 teaspoons cornstarch
1 teaspoon honey
½ teaspoon red
   pepper flakes
¼ teaspoon ground ginger
2 teaspoons sesame oil
4 teaspoons minced garlic
12 ounces raw shrimp
   (31 to 35 count)
¼ cup sliced scallions
1 tablespoon
   sesame seeds
1 cup shredded or
   matchstick-cut carrots

1 To make the zoodles, cut off the ends of the zucchini, and then use a mandolin, spiralizer, or the side of a box grater to cut the zucchini into long, thin strips.

2 In a medium skillet over medium heat, heat the olive oil. Add the zucchini strips, and sauté for 5 minutes, or until tender. Transfer to a bowl and set aside.

3 In a small bowl, make the sauce by whisking together the water, catsup, soy sauce, cornstarch, honey, red pepper flakes, and ginger.

4 Place the same skillet used to cook the zucchini noodles over medium heat, and add the sesame oil. Add the garlic and sauté for 30 seconds to 1 minute, until fragrant. Add the shrimp, and sauté for about 1 minute. Add the scallions and sesame seeds, and sauté for about 3 minutes more, or until the shrimp turn pink.

5 Pour the sauce into the skillet, and continue cooking until the sauce thickens and begins to simmer, about 3 minutes.

6 Remove the skillet from the heat, and stir in the carrots.

7 Serve the shrimp and sauce over the zoodles.

Ingredient tip: *Buy precooked, tail-off shrimp to save time.*

Per Serving (1 cup): Calories: 121 Total fat: 5g Sodium: 572mg
Total carbs: 9g Sugar: 4g Fiber: 2g Protein: 10g

Post-Op Servings

Ⓖ 1 cup

Easy Shrimp Cocktail

MAKES ABOUT 16 SHRIMP / PREP: 10 MINUTES / COOK: 5 MINUTES / TOTAL: 15 MINUTES

With fried foods out of the question, the post-op diet is an opportunity to venture into trying more baked, boiled, and grilled seafood. A recipe for shrimp cocktail seems so simple, yet it's an opportunity for perfect preparation of this shellfish—especially for the kitchen novice. These boiled shrimp are so flavorful you can toss them on top of a salad, serve them over sautéed vegetables, or eat solo to get your protein fix.

1 lemon, halved
   and seeded

1 tablespoon black
   peppercorns

1 teaspoon dried thyme

1 dried bay leaf

½ pound raw shrimp
   (31 to 35 count)

¼ cup Seafood Sauce
   (page 169)

1 Fill a large pot with water. Squeeze the juice from the lemon halves into the water, and add the black peppercorns, thyme, and bay leaf. Place the pot over high heat, and bring to a boil.

2 While the water is heating, create an ice bath by filling a large bowl with ice and water and set aside.

3 Add the shrimp to the boiling water, and cook them for 2 to 3 minutes, or until they just turn pink.

4 Drain the shrimp in a colander and immediately put them in the ice bath to cool.

5 Peel the shrimp and remove the tails. Serve over ice with a dish of the seafood sauce.

Post-Op Servings

Ⓟ 4 shrimp pureed with 1 tablespoon Seafood Sauce

Ⓖ 8 shrimp (4 ounces) with 2 tablespoons Seafood Sauce

Did you know? *Shellfish get a bad rap for being high in cholesterol—but research shows the cholesterol in seafood does not significantly raise blood cholesterol levels. Seafood is virtually fat-free with the exception of heart-healthy omega-3 fats.*

Per Serving (4 shrimp with 1 tablespoon sauce): Calories: 65 Total fat: 1g Sodium: 550mg Total carbs: 6g Sugar: 3g Fiber: 0g Protein: 8g

Classic Crab-Stuffed Tomatoes

SERVES 4 / PREP: 10 MINUTES / TOTAL: 10 MINUTES

Your picnics will never be the same with these crab-stuffed tomatoes. This recipe skips the typical high-fat versions with carb-heavy pasta in exchange for creamy crab salad stuffed inside a juicy, fresh tomato. Make sure to take one for yourself first, because they will disappear fast.

4 medium Roma
   tomatoes
1 cup lump crabmeat or
   1 (6-ounce) can
   crabmeat, drained
1 tablespoon olive oil
   mayonnaise
1 tablespoon low-fat plain
   Greek yogurt
1 tablespoon chopped
   fresh basil
1 teaspoon Dijon mustard
½ teaspoon freshly
   squeezed lemon juice
½ teaspoon hot sauce
   (optional)
2 tablespoons sliced
   scallions

1 Carefully cut off the top of each tomato, and scoop out the pulp and seeds from inside. Discard or save the pulp for use in soups, stews, and chili.

2 In a medium bowl, mix together the crabmeat, mayonnaise, yogurt, basil, mustard, lemon juice, and hot sauce (if using).

3 Gently fill each tomato with the crab salad mixture, and top each with the chopped scallions.

4 Chill until ready to serve.

Ingredient tip: *This is a great recipe to puree during the early post-op period. To boost protein content, puree the crab salad without the tomato, and mix in 1 tablespoon of unflavored protein powder or egg white powder.*

Per Serving (1 stuffed tomato): Calories: 94 Total fat: 2g
Sodium: 229mg Total carbs: 9g Sugar: 4g Fiber: 2g Protein: 10g

Post-Op Servings

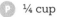

P ¼ cup

S ½ cup (no tomato)

G 1 stuffed tomato

Tuna Noodle-less Casserole

SERVES 10 / PREP: 15 MINUTES / COOK: 40 MINUTES / TOTAL: 55 MINUTES

Tuna noodle casserole is a classic comfort meal that's quick to prepare for a weeknight meal, and it provides an easy way to sneak fish into everyone's diet. I always keep the ingredients on hand in my cupboard for a last-minute meal on those extra-busy days. This recipe is so creamy, flavorful, and delicious you won't even know the noodles are missing. The red bell peppers, tomatoes, and green beans give it just a bit of color to make it more interesting than the typical boring beige version.

Nonstick cooking spray

1 medium red onion, chopped

1 red bell pepper, chopped

1½ cups diced tomato

3 cups fresh green beans

⅓ cup olive oil mayonnaise

1 recipe Homemade Condensed Cream of Mushroom Soup (page 170)

½ cup low-fat milk

1 cup shredded Cheddar cheese

Freshly ground black pepper

3 (5-ounce) cans water-packed albacore tuna, drained

1 Preheat the oven to 425°F.

2 Coat a large skillet with cooking spray, and place it over medium heat.

3 Add the onion, red bell pepper, and tomato, and sauté for 5 minutes, or until the vegetables are tender and the tomato starts to soften. Remove the skillet from the heat and set aside.

4 Cut off the stem ends of the green beans, and snap them into 3- to 4-inch pieces.

5 Fill a large saucepot one-third full with water, and place a steamer basket inside. Place the pot over high heat, and bring the water to a boil.

6 Add the green beans to the steamer basket, cover the pot, and turn down the heat to medium. Steam the green beans for 5 minutes. Immediately remove them from the heat, drain, and set aside.

7 Coat a 9-by-13-inch casserole dish with cooking spray.

8 In a large bowl, mix together the mayonnaise, condensed soup, milk, and cheese. Season the mixture with up to ½ teaspoon of black pepper.

9 Add the tuna, green beans, and sautéed vegetables to the bowl, and mix to combine. Pour the mixture into the casserole dish.

10 Bake for 30 minutes, or until the edges start to brown, and serve.

Ingredient tip: *Choose canned or packets of tuna packed in water instead of oil to save on calories without sacrificing protein. Tuna is an excellent source of not only anti-inflammatory omega-3 fatty acids and protein but also selenium, which is an important mineral and antioxidant.*

Per Serving (1 cup): Calories: 147 Total fat: 7g Sodium: 318mg
Total carbs: 6g Sugar: 2g Fiber: 2g Protein: 15g

Post-Op Servings

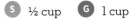 S ½ cup   G 1 cup

Peggy's Salmon Cakes

SERVES 4 / PREP: 15 MINUTES / COOK: 10 MINUTES / TOTAL: 25 MINUTES

These salmon patties are tender and delicious. They can be mixed together ahead of time and baked the day of serving. Try topping them with a dill sauce made from low-fat plain Greek yogurt mixed with dried dill and garlic. As your post-op diet progresses, serve these salmon cakes with mixed vegetables and a small amount of a cooked grain, like protein-packed quinoa or high-fiber barley.

1 (14.75-ounce) can wild pink salmon, drained

½ cup saltine cracker crumbs

2 eggs, lightly beaten

½ teaspoon salt

⅛ teaspoon ground paprika

½ teaspoon dried dill

½ teaspoon parsley flakes

1 Preheat the oven to 375°F.

2 In medium bowl, use clean hands to mix together the salmon, cracker crumbs, eggs, salt, paprika, dill, and parsley flakes until well combined.

3 Form the salmon mixture into 4 patties, and place on an ungreased 9-by-13-inch rimmed baking sheet.

4 Bake for 10 minutes, flipping the cakes over once after 5 minutes.

5 The salmon cakes are done when slightly browned on top. Serve immediately.

Post-Op Servings

S ½ salmon patty

G 1 salmon patty

Did you know? *Salmon is a superfood. It's well known for its high content of omega-3 fatty acids—important for not only heart but brain health as well. Additionally, salmon is a great source of vitamin D. Vitamin D is normally made in our skin from the sun during peak hours of the day and year, but it's very difficult to get from dietary sources. People who struggle with obesity are at high risk for vitamin D deficiency, and most are advised to take a supplement.*

Per Serving (1 patty): Calories: 145 Total fat: 5g Sodium: 638mg
Total carbs: 7g Sugar: 0g Fiber: 0g Protein: 18g

Baked Salmon with Barbecue Seasoning

SERVES 2 / PREP: 10 MINUTES / COOK: 20 MINUTES / TOTAL: 30 MINUTES

Salmon is one of the top power foods for your entire body. It's packed with heart-healthy omega-3 fatty acids, which have amazing anti-inflammatory properties in the body. Salmon contains just as much protein as chicken or beef, but with only healthy fats. Leftover salmon is great scrambled with eggs or tossed in with a green salad.

2 (4-ounce) salmon fillets

1 tablespoon maple syrup

Juice of ½ lemon

1½ teaspoons Chili Powder (page 175)

1½ teaspoons dried paprika

½ teaspoon garlic powder

Post-Op Servings

(S) 2 ounces

(G) 4 ounces

1 Preheat the oven to 400°F. Line a baking dish or rimmed baking sheet with aluminum foil.

2 Place the salmon skin-side down in the dish.

3 Pour the maple syrup and lemon juice over the salmon.

4 Sprinkle the chili powder, paprika, and garlic powder over the fillets.

5 Bake for 20 minutes. The salmon is done when the fish flakes easily with a fork.

6 Serve immediately.

Ingredient tip: *Don't overcook the salmon. Overcooked fish turns rubbery, and the "fishy" flavor tends to be emphasized. Fish is safely cooked when the internal temperature measures 145°F with a meat thermometer.*

Per Serving (4 ounces): Calories: 197 Total fat: 8g Sodium: 53mg Total carbs: 9g Sugar: 7g Fiber: 0g Protein: 23g

Tilapia Tacos with Red Cabbage

SERVES 4 / PREP: 10 MINUTES / COOK: 5 MINUTES / TOTAL: 15 MINUTES

Fish tacos are a popular item at many Tex-Mex restaurants, but as the fish is typically deep-fried and the creamy dressing is high in fat, they become a meal of the past after weight-loss surgery. But fear not. Check out this recipe for flavorful tilapia tacos you can make at home with a spicy seasoning so delicious, the deep-fried version becomes a distant memory. Use Avocado-Lime Dressing (page 166) for a creamy topping without the excessive calories and saturated fat.

4 (4-ounce) tilapia fillets

1 tablespoon extra-virgin olive oil, plus additional for brushing the fish

1 tablespoon Cajun Seasoning (page 174)

4 (7- to 8-inch) whole-wheat tortillas, such as La Tortilla Factory low-carb tortillas

¾ cup shredded red cabbage

2 limes, quartered

¼ cup Avocado-Lime Dressing (page 166) or 1 avocado, sliced

Post-Op Servings

Ⓢ 2 ounces tilapia (no cabbage or tortilla)

Ⓖ 1 taco with 4 ounces tilapia

1 Rinse the tilapia fillets under cold water and pat dry with a paper towel.

2 Brush the fillets lightly with olive oil using a pastry or marinade brush.

3 Sprinkle the fillets on both sides with the Cajun seasoning and set aside.

4 In a large skillet over medium heat, heat 1 tablespoon of olive oil. Once the oil is hot, add the fish, cook for 2 minutes, and then flip the fillets over and continue cooking for 2 minutes more, or until the fish begins to flake.

5 Transfer the fish to a plate or cutting board and cut the fillets into 2-inch chunks. You can use a fork to do this since the fish should fall apart and flake easily.

6 Warm the tortillas for 10 to 15 seconds in the microwave.

7 Prepare the tacos by filling each tortilla with tilapia chunks and red cabbage. Squeeze the juice of the lime wedges over each taco, top with the dressing, and serve.

Per Serving (1 taco): Calories: 242 Total fat: 10g Sodium: 365mg Total carbs: 16g Sugar: 1g Fiber: 8g Protein: 32g

Crispy Baked Cod

SERVES 6 / PREP: 10 MINUTES / COOK: 10 MINUTES / TOTAL: 20 MINUTES

Alas, fried fish dinners are no more. But just because you've given up fried foods doesn't mean you can't have a crispy, well-seasoned fish dinner that doesn't taste a thing like "diet" food. For an extra pop of tartness, finish with freshly squeezed lemon juice and serve with a side of roasted vegetables.

Nonstick cooking spray

6 (4-ounce) skinless
cod fillets

¾ teaspoon salt

¼ teaspoon freshly
ground black pepper

3 tablespoons extra-virgin
olive oil, divided

Juice of 1 lemon, divided

¼ cup dried whole-wheat
bread crumbs

3 tablespoons chopped
fresh parsley

2 tablespoons
chopped chives

Post-Op Servings

Ⓢ 2 to 4 ounces

Ⓖ 4 ounces

1 Preheat the oven to 425°F. Coat a 9-by-13-inch baking dish with cooking spray.

2 Season the cod fillets on both sides with the salt and pepper and arrange in the baking dish so that they do not overlap each other. Drizzle the fish with 1½ tablespoons of olive oil and half the lemon juice.

3 In a small bowl, mix to combine the bread crumbs, parsley, and chives. Sprinkle the mixture over the fillets, and then drizzle them with the remaining 1½ tablespoons of olive oil and lemon juice.

4 Bake the fillets until the bread crumbs are crisp and the cod flakes easily with a fork, about 12 minutes, and serve.

Ingredient tip: *Fish is easily digested and generally well tolerated after surgery, more so than poultry, pork, or beef. You can use any type of hearty white fish for this recipe, such as Alaskan pollock, grouper, haddock, halibut, or swordfish.*

Per Serving (4 ounces): Calories: 165 Total fat: 8g Sodium: 411mg
Total carbs: 5g Sugar: 1g Fiber: 0g Protein: 18g

Grilled Honey Mustard Salmon

SERVES 3 / PREP: 10 MINUTES, PLUS 30 MINUTES TO 2 HOURS TO MARINATE /
COOK: 10 MINUTES / TOTAL: 50 MINUTES AT MINIMUM

Grilling is a favorite meal preparation method of many household chefs, and it doesn't have to be abandoned just because you aren't eating burgers, sausages, and ribs any longer. Grilling is a great method to prepare lean and flavorful proteins. This grilled salmon has a sweet and savory marinade, which will tantalize your taste buds. Turn up the grill and look out—the sweet smell might even bring the neighbors over.

1½ tablespoons honey

2 tablespoons rice
   wine vinegar

2 teaspoons minced garlic

2 teaspoons
   Dijon mustard

2 teaspoons extra-virgin
   olive oil

Juice of ½ lemon

¼ teaspoon freshly
   ground black pepper

¼ teaspoon ground
   cayenne pepper

3 (4-ounce) salmon fillets,
   fresh or frozen, thawed

1 In a small bowl, whisk together the honey, vinegar, garlic, mustard, olive oil, lemon juice, black pepper, and cayenne pepper.

2 Put the salmon in a large zip-top bag, and pour the marinade into the bag. Shake the bag to coat the salmon in the marinade. Seal the bag and refrigerate for 30 minutes to 2 hours.

3 While the salmon marinates, preheat the grill to medium heat, or prepare a charcoal grill. Lightly oil the grill grate so the fish won't stick as it cooks.

4 Place the salmon skin-side down on the grill and cook for about 8 minutes, until the fish flakes easily with a fork or reaches an internal temperature of 145°F, and serve.

Post-Op Servings

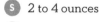

S 2 to 4 ounces

G 4 ounces

Serving tip: *Serve this fish with steamed lentils and sautéed cherry tomatoes, spinach, and leeks. Look for precooked bags of steamed lentils in the produce section of the grocery store; they just need to be reheated before serving. Sauté the vegetables for 5 to 8 minutes in 1 teaspoon of extra-virgin olive oil to soften the leeks and tomatoes and wilt the spinach.*

Per Serving (4 ounces): Calories: 174 Total fat: 4g Sodium: 151mg
Total carbs: 13g Sugar: 9g Fiber: 0g Protein: 25g

Halibut with Cilantro, Lime, and Garlic

SERVES 3 / PREP: 10 MINUTES / COOK: 15 MINUTES / TOTAL: 25 MINUTES

Dreaming of a vacation in warm weather, maybe lying on the beach in Mexico? This cilantro-lime halibut will have you feeling like you are right in the Caribbean—with a swimsuit-ready body in no time. This halibut is so low in calories and rich in protein, it's a perfect meal as a part of your weight-loss plan.

Nonstick cooking spray

3 (4-ounce) halibut fillets

½ cup white wine

¼ cup chopped fresh cilantro

Juice of 1 lime

1 tablespoon extra-virgin olive oil

2 teaspoons minced garlic

Post-Op Servings

(S) 2 to 4 ounces

(G) 4 ounces

1 Preheat the oven to 400°F. Coat a 9-by-13-inch baking dish with cooking spray.

2 Place the halibut fillets in the baking dish.

3 In a small bowl, whisk together the wine, cilantro, lime juice, olive oil, and garlic. Pour this dressing over the fillets.

4 Bake for 12 to 15 minutes, or until the fish flakes easily with a fork, and serve.

Per Serving (4 ounces): Calories: 177 Total fat: 6g Sodium: 80mg Total carbs: 1g Sugar: 0g Fiber: 0g Protein: 21g

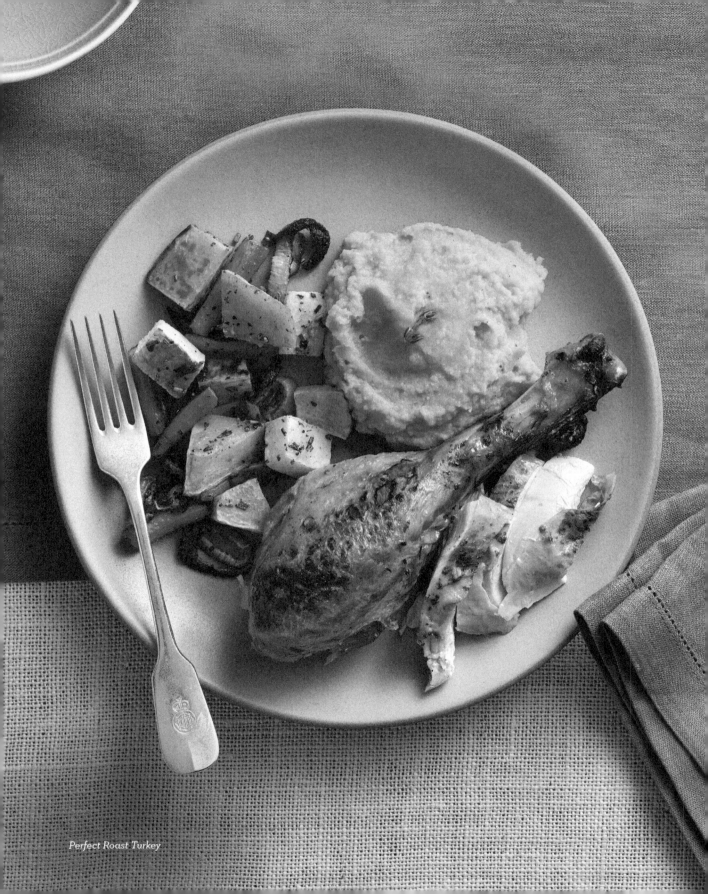

Perfect Roast Turkey

Poultry Dinners

Slow Cooker Chicken Taco Soup

SERVES 10
PREP: 15 MINUTES / COOK: 8 HOURS, 20 MINUTES / TOTAL: 8 HOURS, 35 MINUTES

Many hearty chicken tortilla soups are made with heavy cream and topped with loads of fried tortilla chips. This version skips those weight loss–adverse ingredients, but is not short on flavor. It is jam-packed with seasoning and is so hearty it will certainly leave you full and satisfied. This is a great recipe to make for a crowd since you can toss it together ahead of time. If you must have the crunchy chips, choose a 100 percent whole-grain chip—ideally a sprouted grain if possible, and limit to a small handful to avoid unnecessary calories.

1½ pounds boneless, skinless chicken breasts

1 (14.5-ounce) can black beans, drained and rinsed

1 (14.5-ounce) can diced tomatoes or 2 cups chopped fresh tomatoes

1 (4.5-ounce) can chopped green chiles

¾ cup chopped onion

1 green bell pepper, chopped into ¼-inch pieces

1 cup chicken broth

½ cup water

4 teaspoons minced garlic

1 tablespoon Chili Powder (page 175)

1 teaspoon ground cumin

½ teaspoon ground coriander

Optional add-ins per bowl

Chopped fresh cilantro

Sliced avocado

Shredded Cheddar cheese

Low-fat plain Greek yogurt

1 Place the chicken breasts in the bottom of a slow cooker. Add the black beans, tomatoes, chiles, onion, and bell pepper.

2 In a small bowl mix together the broth, water, garlic, chili powder, cumin, and coriander. Pour the mixture over the chicken and vegetables in the slow cooker.

3 Cover and cook on low for 7 to 8 hours.

4 Prior to serving, transfer the chicken to a plate and shred it with a fork. Return it to the slow cooker for an additional 20 minutes so the meat can absorb some of the soup.

5 To serve, garnish each bowl with the cilantro, avocado, cheese, and yogurt (if using).

Per Serving (1 cup without add-ins): Calories: 125 Total fat: 1g Sodium: 583mg Total carbs: 11g Sugar: 2g Fiber: 4g Protein: 18g

Post-Op Servings

P ¼ cup   S ½ cup   G 1 cup

Chicken Caesar Wraps with Kale

MAKES 5 WRAPS / PREP: 15 MINUTES / TOTAL: 15 MINUTES

Wraps make good alternatives to sandwiches for lunch since many post-op patients cannot tolerate the doughy bread in a sandwich. Plus you can find many wraps that are low in calories and carbohydrates. Most low-calorie wraps (the wrap itself, not including what you put in it) come in at 90 calories or less, which is the equivalent of 1 slice of bread. Try this twist on a Caesar wrap with kale—the dressing helps reduce the sometimes bitter taste of kale. You can always make this a "naked" wrap and do without the outer shell.

3 cups cooked chicken breast—grilled and sliced, canned, or shredded rotisserie chicken

1 cup chopped romaine lettuce

1 cup chopped kale leaves

¾ cup Low-Fat Caesar Dressing (page 167)

¼ cup shredded Parmesan cheese

3 tablespoons sunflower seeds

5 small 100 percent whole-grain low-carb wraps, such as Tumaro's low-carb wraps

Post-Op Servings

G 1 wrap

1 In a large mixing bowl, mix to combine the chicken, romaine, kale, dressing, cheese, and sunflower seeds. If you are concerned the kale is too tough, try mixing it with ¼ cup of dressing 30 minutes prior to mixing it with the other ingredients to help soften the leaves.

2 Place about 1 cup of the salad mixture onto each wrap. Fold the wrap over the top of the salad, close in the sides, and then tightly roll the wrap closed. Use a toothpick to secure the wrap if needed and serve.

Ingredient tip: *Packed with vitamin C, iron, and folate, kale is one of the most nutrient-dense greens you can eat. No worries if your family is stuck on eating iceberg lettuce and kale seems like a long way away—take baby steps. Try transitioning from iceberg lettuce to romaine lettuce. Then move on to spinach and eventually try kale. By transitioning slowly to stronger-flavored greens, you won't taste the difference as much, and before you know it you will be including these power-packed greens on a daily basis.*

Per Serving (1 wrap): Calories: 332 Total fat: 13g Sodium: 447mg Total carbs: 17g Sugar: 1g Fiber: 9g Protein: 36g

Chicken Asian Lettuce Wraps

MAKES 8 WRAPS / PREP: 15 MINUTES / COOK: 10 MINUTES / TOTAL: 25 MINUTES

These lettuce wraps rival those at P. F. Chang's but have far fewer calories and much less sodium. Lettuce wraps make an amazing and delicious appetizer, or serve them as a quick meal. They are packed with protein and flavor and are low in carbohydrates. Chinese food craving solved!

1 (8-ounce) can bamboo shoots, drained and minced

3 tablespoons apple cider vinegar

1 tablespoon creamy natural peanut butter

2 teaspoons low-sodium soy sauce or Bragg Liquid Aminos

2 teaspoons sriracha hot sauce

2 teaspoons honey

Nonstick cooking spray

1 cup chopped onion

1 tablespoon minced garlic

½ pound ground chicken breast

1 teaspoon minced ginger

1 teaspoon sesame oil

8 leaves iceberg or butter lettuce

1 scallion, chopped

1 small cucumber, cut into strips

1　In a small bowl, mix together the bamboo shoots, apple cider vinegar, peanut butter, soy sauce, sriracha, and honey until well combined.

2　Place a medium skillet over medium heat and coat with cooking spray. Add the onion and garlic, and sauté until the onion is soft, 3 to 4 minutes.

3　Add the ground chicken and ginger, and cook until the chicken is no longer pink, about 5 minutes.

4　Stir in the sauce mixture and continue cooking for 2 minutes, or until heated through. Stir in the sesame oil.

5　Remove the skillet from the heat, and divide the mixture evenly among the lettuce leaves.

6　Top each wrap with some scallion and cucumber and serve immediately.

Per Serving (1 wrap): Calories: 88 Total fat: 4g Sodium: 95mg Total carbs: 5g Sugar: 2g Fiber: 1g Protein: 8g

Post-Op Servings

Ⓖ 2 wraps

Spicy Chicken Stuffed with Spinach and Cheese

SERVES 4 / PREP: 15 MINUTES / COOK: 40 MINUTES / TOTAL: 55 MINUTES

This chicken is sure to excite your taste buds, and it's a lean replacement for spicy fried wings. Don't concern yourself with getting the roll-ups perfect. Either way, they will still turn out tender and delicious. And you can spoon any leftover cheesy spinach that may have bubbled over during cooking right on top.

Nonstick cooking spray

4 (4-ounce) boneless, skinless chicken breasts

4 ounces pepper Jack cheese, shredded

1 cup cooked spinach (steam 2 to 3 cups fresh spinach in the microwave for 2 minutes)

1¾ tablespoons Cajun Seasoning (page 174)

2 tablespoons whole-wheat bread crumbs

2 teaspoons extra-virgin olive oil

Post-Op Servings

Ⓖ 1 stuffed chicken breast

1 Preheat the oven to 350°F degrees. Coat a 9-by-13-inch baking dish with cooking spray and set aside.

2 Using a meat tenderizing mallet, flatten the chicken breasts to ¼-inch thickness. Set aside.

3 In a small bowl, mix together the cheese and cooked spinach.

4 In another small bowl, mix to combine the Cajun seasoning and bread crumbs.

5 Spoon about 2 tablespoons of the cheese and spinach mixture onto each chicken breast. Roll up each chicken breast, and secure with one or two toothpicks.

6 Place the chicken seam-side up in the baking dish.

7 Using a pastry or marinade brush, brush each chicken roll-up with the olive oil. Sprinkle the seasoned bread crumbs over each roll-up.

8 Bake for 35 to 40 minutes, or until the chicken juices run clear and the topping begins to brown. Serve immediately.

Per Serving (1 chicken roll-up): Calories: 241 Total fat: 10g
Sodium: 453mg Total carbs: 2g Sugar: 0g Fiber: 1g Protein: 32g

Baked Garlic–Greek Yogurt Chicken with Parmesan

SERVES 4 / PREP: 10 MINUTES / COOK: 45 MINUTES / TOTAL: 55 MINUTES

Chicken breast is a go-to meal for many patients post-op since it's easy, low in calories, and inexpensive to make. This recipe is a twist on the traditional version, which is coated in heavy full-fat mayo. The Greek yogurt coating traps in moisture to keep the chicken juicy and tender.

Nonstick cooking spray

1 cup low-fat plain
   Greek yogurt

½ cup shredded
   Parmesan cheese

1½ teaspoons
   seasoning salt

1 teaspoon garlic powder

½ teaspoon freshly
   ground black pepper

4 (4-ounce) boneless,
   skinless chicken breasts

1 Preheat the oven to 375°F. Coat a 9-by-13-inch baking dish with cooking spray and set aside.

2 In a small bowl, mix to combine the yogurt, cheese, salt, garlic powder, and pepper.

3 Place the chicken breasts in the baking dish.

4 Use a pastry or marinade brush to coat each breast with the yogurt mixture.

5 Bake for 45 minutes, or until the juices run clear and the topping begins to brown, and serve.

Per Serving (1 chicken breast): Calories: 273 Total fat: 8g
Sodium: 519mg Total carbs: 3g Sugar: 2g Fiber: 0g Protein: 45g

Post-Op Servings

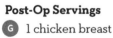 1 chicken breast

Tender Slow Cooker Chicken Tikka Masala

SERVES 10 / PREP: 15 MINUTES / COOK: 4 TO 8 HOURS / TOTAL: 4 TO 8 HOURS

Culinary delights from around the world are increasingly part of the typical American diet. Many are low calorie and healthy, while others are often prepared with high-fat ingredients like butter, cream, and lots of added sodium. This healthier twist on a popular Indian dish is sure to leave you feeling full and satisfied. The creamy tomato sauce is divine and keeps the chicken tender. With the addition of some simple seasonings, you can take a weeknight meal to a whole new level of flavor.

3 pounds boneless, skinless chicken breasts

1 large white onion, diced

2 tablespoons minced ginger or 1½ tablespoons ground ginger

1 (29-ounce) can tomato puree

1½ cups low-fat plain Greek yogurt, plus

additional for garnish (optional)

2 tablespoons garam masala

4 teaspoons minced garlic

1 tablespoon ground cumin

2 teaspoons ground cayenne pepper

1½ teaspoons ground paprika

¾ teaspoon ground cinnamon

¾ teaspoon freshly ground black pepper

2 dried bay leaves

Chopped fresh cilantro, for garnish (optional)

1 In the slow cooker, stir to combine the chicken, onion, ginger, tomato puree, yogurt, garam masala, garlic, cumin, cayenne pepper, paprika, cinnamon, and black pepper, coating the chicken breasts well.

2 Place the bay leaves on top of the mixture.

3 Cover and cook for 4 hours on high or 8 hours on low.

4 Remove the bay leaves. Stir the tikka masala with a wooden spoon, breaking up the chicken breasts. They should break apart easily.

5 Serve each portion garnished with a dollop of yogurt (if using) and a sprinkle of cilantro (if using).

Serving tip: *This low-carb dish is great all on its own, or, if tolerated, you can serve it over brown jasmine rice. Even better, try it over no-carb riced cauliflower. Don't forget the dollop of Greek yogurt on top for additional creaminess and protein.*

Per Serving (5 ounces): Calories: 207 Total fat: 3g Sodium: 622mg Total carbs: 12g Sugar: 5g Fiber: 2g Protein: 33.g

Post-Op Servings

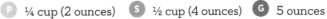

Ⓟ ¼ cup (2 ounces)   Ⓢ ½ cup (4 ounces)   Ⓖ 5 ounces

Creamy Slow Cooker Chicken Breast with Italian Seasonings

SERVES 8 / PREP: 10 MINUTES / COOK: 4 TO 7 HOURS / TOTAL: 4 TO 7 HOURS

Dry foods are not generally well tolerated after surgery. Patients report that if they try to eat meats that are dried out and tough, they feel the food gets stuck and they're unable to eat more than a bite or two. Foods that are moist and have sauces tend to be tolerated best since they can be digested more smoothly—especially during the first few weeks and months post-op. Try this creamy chicken made with Greek yogurt for a meal both you and your waistline will enjoy.

Nonstick cooking spray

6 boneless, skinless chicken breasts (2½ pounds total)

1 recipe Homemade Condensed Cream of Mushroom Soup (page 170)

8 ounces (2½ cups) sliced mushrooms

1 cup low-fat plain Greek yogurt

½ cup chicken broth

2 teaspoons dried oregano

1½ teaspoons garlic powder

1½ teaspoons onion powder

1 teaspoon dried parsley

½ teaspoon freshly ground black pepper

¼ teaspoon dried thyme

¼ teaspoon dried basil

1 Coat the inside of a slow cooker with cooking spray.

2 Place the chicken breasts in the slow cooker.

3 Pour in the mushroom soup, mushrooms, yogurt, broth, oregano, garlic powder, onion powder, parsley, pepper, thyme, and basil. Mix well.

4 Cover the slow cooker and cook on high for 4 hours or on low for 7 hours. Keep warm until ready to serve.

Serving tip: *To keep this meal low carb, eat this chicken without any starchy side dishes. If you are 3 months or more post-op, you can try serving it over boiled potatoes.*

Per Serving (5 ounces meat and 1 ounce sauce): Calories: 206 Total fat: 6g Sodium: 79mg Total carbs: 5g Sugar: 0g Fiber: 1g Protein: 33g

Post-Op Servings

(P) ¼ cup (2 ounces)

(S) ½ cup (4 ounces)

(G) 4 to 6 ounces

Slow Cooker Shredded Chicken for Tacos

SERVES 4 / PREP: 5 MINUTES / COOK: 6 TO 8 HOURS, 30 MINUTES / TOTAL: 6 TO 8 HOURS, 30 MINUTES

Tuesdays are for tacos, but tacos make a quick and easy meal for any weeknight, not to mention that they are also great to serve a crowd on the weekends. Versatility is a bonus, too. You can use this seasoned meat as a topping for salads, inside enchiladas, to make a quick soup or chili, and, of course, as a filling for classic tacos. This meat stores and freezes well for later use. So, it's a matter of when, not if.

4 (4-ounce) boneless, skinless chicken breasts

1¼ cups chicken broth

3 tablespoons Taco Seasoning (page 174)

Post-Op Servings

P ¼ cup (2 ounces)

S ½ cup (4 ounces)

G 4 ounces

1 Place the chicken breasts in the bottom of a slow cooker. Pour the broth and taco seasoning over the chicken.

2 Cover the slow cooker, and cook on low for 6 to 8 hours.

3 Transfer the chicken to a plate and shred it with a fork. Return it to the slow cooker, and cook on low for an additional 30 minutes before serving, allowing the chicken to absorb the liquid.

Serving tip: *How to make the healthiest tacos of the bunch? Use 100 percent whole-grain shells—get the 6- to 7-inch shells versus the 10-inch shells to keep portion size down. Top each taco with Fresh Salsa (page 172), sliced avocado, onions or scallions, bell peppers, black olives, and a bit of shredded lettuce. Or try fresh spinach rather than lettuce to increase the power-food factor. I always put beans in my tacos—Pinto Beans and Cheese (page 40) or black beans to add fiber and more protein.*

Per Serving (4 ounces): Calories: 124 Total fat: 2g Sodium: 719mg
Total carbs: 0g Sugar: 0g Fiber: 0g Protein: 27g

Baked Chimichangas with Chicken and Fresh Salsa

SERVES 6 / PREP: 15 MINUTES / COOK: 25 MINUTES / TOTAL: 40 MINUTES

The deep-fried Tex-Mex burrito—a chimichanga—is a popular item in many Mexican restaurants. With the deep-frying comes a very high fat content, so it's no longer an option after surgery. These baked chimichangas, however, are easy to make at home and satisfy all your cravings for those original ooey gooey deep-fried burritos. Yes, please.

1½ cups chopped cooked chicken

1 cup shredded cheese, such as Colby Jack or Mexican cheese blend

⅔ cup Fresh Salsa (page 172), plus additional for topping

1 teaspoon ground cumin

½ teaspoon dried oregano

¼ teaspoon crushed red pepper

2 scallions, chopped

6 (7- to 8-inch) whole-wheat tortillas, such as La Tortilla Factory low-carb tortillas

2 tablespoons extra-virgin olive oil

1   Preheat the oven to 400°F. Line a large rimmed baking sheet with aluminum foil.

2   In a large bowl, mix together the chicken, cheese, salsa, cumin, oregano, red pepper, and scallions.

3   On a large plate or cutting board, place about ¼ cup of filling mixture in the middle of each tortilla. Fold over the tortilla, pull in the sides, and tightly roll it closed. Place the chimichangas seam-side down on the baking sheet.

4   Using a pastry or marinade brush, lightly brush the top of each chimichanga with the olive oil.

5   Bake for 25 minutes, or until the tops turn golden brown.

6   Garnish each chimichanga with additional salsa before serving.

Per Serving (1 chimichanga): Calories: 205 Total fat: 10g
Sodium: 382mg Total carbs: 13g Sugar: 1g Fiber: 8g Protein: 24g

Post-Op Servings

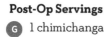 (G) 1 chimichanga

One-Pan Chicken and Broccoli

SERVES 8 / PREP: 10 MINUTES / COOK: 20 MINUTES / TOTAL: 30 MINUTES

Enjoy this quick weeknight meal that the entire family will love. Added bonus: It's as easy to clean up afterward as it is to make because you really only need one pan to whip up this dish. Leftovers are great reheated for a meal later in the week. If you find you're in a time crunch, you can even use meat from a rotisserie chicken to save time.

1 tablespoon extra-virgin olive oil

1 yellow onion, chopped

2 teaspoons minced garlic

1 pound boneless, skinless chicken breast, cooked and diced

1 cup water

1 cup chicken broth

1 cup quinoa

½ teaspoon dried thyme

2½ cups chopped broccoli

1 In a medium skillet over medium heat, heat the olive oil. Add the onion and garlic, and sauté until the onion is soft, 2 to 3 minutes.

2 Add the chicken, water, broth, quinoa, and thyme. Bring the liquid to a boil, cover, reduce the heat to medium-low, and cook for 10 minutes.

3 Add the broccoli, cover, and cook for 7 minutes more, until the quinoa fluffs with a fork and the broccoli is tender.

Did you know? *Quinoa is a gluten-free grain. It is packed with protein, fiber, and lots of B vitamins. Gluten-free does not mean carbohydrate-free or low calorie, but for people who are intolerant to the gluten protein found in wheat, rye, and barley, quinoa is an acceptable alternative.*

Post-Op Servings

Ⓖ 1 cup

Per Serving (1 cup): Calories: 176 Total fat: 4g Sodium: 323mg
Total carbs: 17g Sugar: 1g Fiber: 3g Protein: 17g

Southwest Zucchini and Chicken

SERVES 8 / PREP: 20 MINUTES / COOK: 20 MINUTES / TOTAL: 40 MINUTES

I love meals where you can just dump together lots of fresh ingredients into one pot and come up with a tasty result, especially when the ingredients are low in carbs but full of flavor. This meal can be cooked in one pan and contains tons of fresh vegetables, Tex-Mex seasonings, and protein-dense chicken as well as beans.

1 tablespoon extra-virgin olive oil

1 large onion, finely chopped

1 tablespoon minced garlic

1 medium red bell pepper, diced

1 medium yellow bell pepper, diced

1 pound boneless, skinless chicken breast, chopped

1 tablespoon ground cumin

1 teaspoon Taco Seasoning (page 174)

1 (14.5-ounce) can black beans, drained and rinsed

1 (14.5-ounce) can diced tomatoes

1 cup frozen or fresh corn kernels

1 large zucchini, halved lengthwise and diced

1 cup shredded Colby cheese

1 cup chopped fresh cilantro

½ cup chopped scallions

1 In a large skillet over medium heat, heat the olive oil. Add the onion, garlic, and red and yellow bell peppers. Sauté the vegetables for about 5 minutes, or until tender.

2 Add the chicken, cumin, and taco seasoning, and stir until the chicken and vegetables are well coated.

3 Stir in the beans, tomatoes, and corn. Bring the mixture to a boil, cover the skillet, and cook for 10 minutes.

4 Add the zucchini and mix well. Cook for 7 minutes more, or until the zucchini is tender.

5 Remove the skillet from the heat, mix in the cheese, cilantro, and scallions, and serve.

Per Serving (1 cup): Calories: 240 Total fat: 8g Sodium: 524mg Total carbs: 21g Sugar: 6g Fiber: 7g Protein: 21g

Post-Op Servings

(G) 1 cup

Baked Fried Chicken Thighs

SERVES 4 / PREP: 10 MINUTES / COOK: 35 MINUTES / TOTAL: 45 MINUTES

Fried chicken is the most popular meal ordered in restaurants in the United States, but it's laden with artery-clogging fat and will certainly not be well tolerated by your new stomach after surgery. Try this tasty baked fried chicken recipe, which is loaded with flavor and has a crunchy coating made from cereal that will make you think it was deep-fried.

Nonstick cooking spray

1 teaspoon ground paprika

½ teaspoon garlic powder

½ teaspoon freshly ground black pepper

½ teaspoon ground cayenne pepper

½ teaspoon dried oregano

4 (5-ounce) boneless, skinless chicken thighs

2 eggs

1 tablespoon water

1 teaspoon Dijon mustard

2½ cups bran flakes

1 Preheat the oven to 400°F. Line a large rimmed baking sheet with aluminum foil, and place it in the oven below a clean oven rack. Spray the clean rack with the cooking spray.

2 In a large zip-top bag, combine the paprika, garlic powder, black pepper, cayenne pepper, and oregano. Add the chicken thighs to the bag, seal the bag, and shake to coat the thighs with the seasonings. Set aside.

3 In a small bowl, lightly whisk together the eggs, water, and mustard.

4 Crush the bran flakes in a large plastic bag.

5 To bread the chicken, dredge the seasoned chicken thighs in the egg mixture, and then put them in the bag of crushed cereal. Shake to coat well.

6 Place the chicken thighs on the clean oven rack, making sure the baking sheet is directly under the chicken to collect any drippings.

7 Bake for 35 minutes, or until the thighs are crispy and reach an internal temperature of 165°F, and serve.

Post-op tip: *Dark-meat chicken is slightly higher in cholesterol and saturated fat than its white-meat counterpart, but don't fear trying the dark meat since it tends to be more moist and tender than chicken breast. After surgery, texture is very important to your ability to tolerate different proteins. Balance out this meal by serving with Mashed Cauliflower (page 72) and your choice of vegetables.*

Per Serving (1 chicken thigh): Calories: 272 Total fat: 8g Sodium: 279mg Total carbs: 15g Sugar: 3g Fiber: 3g Protein: 35g

Post-Op Servings

(S) ½ chicken thigh (2 to 4 ounces)

(G) 1 chicken thigh (4 to 6 ounces)

Ground Turkey–Stuffed Acorn Squash with Cheese

SERVES 4 / PREP: 10 MINUTES / COOK: 40 MINUTES / TOTAL: 50 MINUTES

Try this great fall meal as an easy and flavorful way to get in both your protein and vegetables. The acorn squash is a great alternative to potatoes or pasta, and it has a slightly sweet flavor and comforting consistency. Impress your friends and family with this easy meal tonight.

2 acorn squash, halved, pulp and seeds removed

1 pound extra-lean ground turkey breast

1 cup diced celery

1 cup chopped onion

1 cup sliced fresh mushrooms

1 (8-ounce) can tomato sauce

1 teaspoon dried basil

1 teaspoon dried oregano

1 teaspoon garlic powder

Pinch freshly ground black pepper

1 cup shredded Cheddar cheese

Post-Op Servings

S ½ cup filling

G 1 stuffed squash half

1 Preheat the oven to 350°F.

2 Place the squash halves cut-side down in a glass baking dish. Microwave the squash for 20 minutes on high, until almost tender.

3 Transfer the squash, cut-side up, to a 9-by-13-inch baking dish or large baking sheet.

4 While the squash is in the microwave, in a large nonstick saucepan over medium heat, brown the ground turkey until cooked through, 7 to 9 minutes.

5 Add the celery and onion, and cook until tender, about 5 minutes.

6 Stir in the mushrooms, tomato sauce, basil, oregano, garlic powder, and pepper.

7 Spoon the mixture into the squash halves, and top each with ¼ cup of cheese. Cover the stuffed squash with aluminum foil.

8 Bake for 15 minutes. Remove the foil and bake for 5 minutes more, or until the cheese bubbles, and serve.

Post-op tip: *If the portion is too large or the squash is too heavy to tolerate, offer this meal to friends and family and save a small portion of the filling for you to eat on the side.*

Per Serving (1 stuffed squash half): Calories: 371 Total fat: 8g Sodium: 585mg Total carbs: 33g Sugar: 5g Fiber: 6g Protein: 38g

Baked Turkey Meatballs

MAKES 12 MEATBALLS / PREP: 15 MINUTES / COOK: 20 MINUTES / TOTAL: 35 MINUTES

No need to forgo all your favorite comfort meals after weight-loss surgery. This healthier version of classic meatballs is packed with nutrition and flavor. Try it in mini individual servings to help keep portions controlled and make it easier for reheating or serving up leftovers. Serve with Roasted Rosemary Sweet Potato Wedges (page 66).

Nonstick cooking spray

1 egg

16 to 20 ounces ground turkey breast

½ cup old-fashioned oats

1 small onion, chopped

2 tablespoons Worcestershire sauce

1 tablespoon tomato paste

1 teaspoon freshly ground black pepper

Post-Op Servings

S 1 meatball

G 2 to 3 meatballs

1 Preheat the oven to 350°F. Coat the cups of a 12-cup muffin tin with cooking spray.

2 In a small bowl, lightly whisk the egg.

3 In a large bowl, mix together the ground turkey, oats, onion, Worcestershire sauce, tomato paste, pepper, and egg.

4 Using clean hands, shape the turkey mixture into 12 equal-size meatballs and place one in each muffin cup.

5 Bake for 20 minutes, or until the meat is cooked thoroughly and a meat thermometer reads 165°F, and serve.

Per Serving (1 meatball): Calories: 81 Total fat: 1g Sodium: 254mg Total carbs: 8g Sugar: 2g Fiber: 0g Protein: 10g

Skinny Turkey and Wild Rice Soup

SERVES 10 / PREP: 10 MINUTES / COOK: 50 MINUTES / TOTAL: 1 HOUR

Use up those Thanksgiving turkey leftovers with this soup, which will warm your soul. This meal will fill you up and leave you satisfied without the extra fat and calories in typical cream soups. For ingredients, you can also use fat-free milk instead of fat-free half-and-half in a pinch.

1 tablespoon extra-virgin olive oil

1 medium onion, chopped

2 carrots, chopped

2 celery stalks, chopped

2 teaspoons minced garlic

4 ounces (1½ cups) mushrooms, chopped

4 cups chicken broth, divided

3 tablespoons whole-wheat pastry flour

2 cups water

1 cup wild rice

1 teaspoon dried thyme

½ teaspoon freshly ground black pepper

1 dried bay leaf

2 cups cooked, shredded or cubed turkey breast

1 cup fat-free half-and-half

1 In a large stockpot over medium heat, heat the olive oil. Add the onion, carrots, celery, and garlic, and sauté until tender, 3 to 4 minutes.

2 Add the mushrooms, and cook for 2 minutes more.

3 Add ½ cup of broth and the flour, and stir until well combined.

4 Stir in the remaining 3½ cups of broth and the water, wild rice, thyme, pepper, and bay leaf. Bring to a boil, cover, reduce the heat to a simmer, and cook for 25 minutes.

5 Stir in the turkey, and continue cooking for 7 minutes.

6 Remove the bay leaf and stir in the half-and-half. Cook for 10 minutes more before serving.

Post-op tip: *Rice is a starchy food that is not always tolerated after surgery. Wait until you are at least 3 months post-op to try this soup. You can always omit the rice from the recipe along with about 2 cups of water and broth and still have a tasty, thick, creamy turkey soup to enjoy.*

Post-Op Servings

Ⓖ 1 cup

Per Serving (1 cup): Calories: 183 Total fat: 3g Sodium: 269mg
Total carbs: 19g Sugar: 3g Fiber: 2g Protein: 20g

Grilled Turkey Burger Patties

MAKES 8 PATTIES / PREP: 10 MINUTES / COOK: 10 MINUTES / TOTAL: 20 MINUTES

Swap beef for lean ground turkey the next time you crave a burger to save on calories and fat. You won't compromise flavor when you mix in cumin, cayenne, oregano, and onion powder. I always mix in a pinch or two of flaxseed—you will never know it's there, but it's a great way to sneak this power food into your diet on a regular basis. These turkey burger patties are so tasty you won't even need to serve them on a bun. Serve them with a mixed green salad with a flavored vinegar for dressing and a side of Roasted Rosemary Sweet Potato Wedges (page 66).

16 ounces extra-lean ground turkey

¼ cup whole-wheat bread crumbs

1 red bell pepper, finely minced

1 egg

1 tablespoon flaxseed

1 teaspoon onion powder

½ teaspoon ground cayenne pepper

½ teaspoon ground cumin

½ teaspoon dried oregano

Post-Op Servings

Ⓖ 2 (2- to 3-ounce) burger patties

1 Prepare an outdoor grill for medium heat.

2 In large mixing bowl, mix together the turkey, bread crumbs, red bell pepper, egg, flaxseed, onion powder, cayenne pepper, cumin, and oregano.

3 Form the mixture into 8 turkey patties, about 3 ounces each.

4 Place the patties on the hottest part of the grill, and grill for 4 minutes. Flip the patties over and grill for another 2 to 3 minutes, or until the meat is cooked through and reaches an internal temperature of 165°F.

5 Let the patties rest for 2 to 3 minutes before serving.

Cooking tip: *Don't have a grill? You can also prepare these patties on the stove. Spray a large nonstick skillet or griddle with nonstick cooking spray, and set over medium heat. Carefully place the burgers in the pan, and cook for 6 minutes. Flip using a large spatula, and continue cooking for 4 minutes on the other side. The patties are finished when they are no longer pink and the internal temperature is at least 165°F.*

Per Serving (2 burger patties): Calories: 189 Total fat: 3g
Sodium: 143mg Total carbs: 9g Sugar: 2g Fiber: 2g Protein: 29g

Perfect Roast Turkey

SERVES 6 / PREP: 15 MINUTES / COOK: 3 HOURS, PLUS 25 MINUTES TO REST / TOTAL: LESS THAN 4 HOURS

Thanksgiving turkey doesn't have to be basted with butter and loaded with sausage stuffing to be delicious. Check out this very simple recipe for making a low-calorie and heart-healthy, buttery, tender turkey. Nor does it have to be reserved for one day out of the year. Make this year-round to serve up a lean source of protein. Leftovers can easily be made into soups and stews and used as a topping for salad.

1 (10-pound) turkey

¾ cup extra-virgin olive oil

1 tablespoon minced garlic

2 teaspoons dried basil

1 teaspoon dried rosemary

1 teaspoon dried sage

½ teaspoon freshly ground black pepper

2 teaspoons ground paprika

About 2 cups water

1 Preheat the oven to 375°F.

2 Remove and discard the neck and giblets from the turkey cavity, and use a paper towel to pat the turkey dry. Place the turkey in a large roasting pan. Tie the legs together with kitchen twine and tuck under the wing tips. Make some cuts in the skin with a sharp knife or kitchen scissors.

3 In a small bowl, mix together the olive oil, garlic, basil, rosemary, sage, and pepper.

4 Use a pastry or marinade brush to coat the outside of the turkey with the mixture, and get as much as possible under the skin.

5 Sprinkle the outside of the turkey with the paprika.

6 Pour the water around (not over) the turkey in the roasting pan. Cover with a lid or aluminum foil tightly.

7 Roast for 3 hours, or until the temperature of the innermost part of a thigh and thickest part of the breast has reached 165°F.

8 Remove the turkey from the oven, and let it rest for 20 to 25 minutes before carving.

Serving tip: *Serve with Roasted Tomatoes, Peppers, and Zucchini with Italian Herbs (page 64), or try roasted carrots, zucchini, and Brussels sprouts. To make a side of pureed sweet potatoes: Toss cooked sweet potatoes into a blender or food processor with ¼ to ½ cup of vegetable or chicken broth and puree until smooth. Make sure to use portion control on any added butter spreads (1 teaspoon at the most).*

Did you know? *Always practice good food safety techniques when thawing raw meat, since it can be a source of harmful bacteria. For a 10-pound turkey, thaw it for 1 to 3 days in the refrigerator ahead of the day you desire to roast it. A more rapid method for thawing is to use a cold water bath. Fill your sink or a very large stockpot with cold water, and thaw the turkey for 2 to 6 hours, changing the water frequently to prevent the growth of harmful bacteria. Make sure to properly clean and sanitize your sink or pot after thawing.*

Per Serving (4 ounces): Calories: 200 Total fat: 8g Sodium: 120mg Total carbs: 0g Sugar: 0g Fiber: 0g Protein: 32g

Post-Op Servings

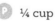 ¼ cup (2 ounces) ⓢ ½ cup (4 ounces) Ⓖ 4 to 6 ounces

Best-Yet Turkey Chili

SERVES 8 / PREP: 10 MINUTES / COOK: 40 MINUTES / TOTAL: 50 MINUTES

This meaty chili is hearty enough to fill you up on a cold winter day but lean enough in calories to help you meet your weight-loss goals. It has a balance of meat and beans that will please everyone in the crowd. The perfect blend of spices from the homemade Chili Powder (page 175) and additional cumin give this chili flavor to delight your palate.

Nonstick cooking spray

16 to 20 ounces extra-lean ground turkey

1 white onion, chopped

1 tablespoon minced garlic

2 cups water

1 (28-ounce) can crushed tomatoes

1 (15-ounce) can red kidney beans, drained and rinsed

2 tablespoons Chili Powder (page 175)

½ teaspoon ground paprika

½ teaspoon dried oregano

½ teaspoon ground cumin

1 Place a large pot over medium-high heat, and coat it with cooking spray. Add the ground turkey, and brown it for about 7 minutes, or until the turkey is no longer pink.

2 Add the onion and garlic to the pot, and sauté until the onion is tender, about 5 minutes.

3 Stir in the water, crushed tomatoes, kidney beans, chili powder, paprika, oregano, and cumin until well combined.

4 Bring the liquid to a simmer, and then turn down the heat to low. Cook for about 30 minutes, until the chili is thick and no longer watery, and serve.

Post-op tip: *You may find this to be a well-tolerated staple during post-op. Add powdered eggs or an unflavored protein powder to get in additional grams of protein. To jazz up the recipe as you advance several months after surgery, top the chili with low-fat plain Greek yogurt, shredded cheese, and chopped scallions. You could even try this poured over a quartered or halved baked potato.*

Per Serving (1 cup): Calories: 141 Total fat: 1g Sodium: 176mg
Total carbs: 15g Sugar: 4g Fiber: 4g Protein: 19g

Post-Op Servings

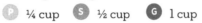

P ¼ cup   S ½ cup   G 1 cup

Beef and
Barley Soup

CHAPTER EIGHT

Pork and Beef Dinners

Zucchini Boats Stuffed with Ground Beef and Cheese

SERVES 8 / PREP: 15 MINUTES / COOK: 30 MINUTES / TOTAL: 45 MINUTES

Here are your Italian favorites packed into one meal—lean ground beef, mozzarella cheese, Italian seasonings, and tomatoes—without the heavy carb-laden pasta. If you garden, this is a great way to use up the plentiful zucchini harvest.

4 medium zucchini

Nonstick cooking spray

1 pound extra-lean
   ground beef

½ cup chopped onion

1 egg, lightly beaten

½ pound mushrooms,
   sliced

1 large tomato, diced

1 (8-ounce) can
   tomato sauce

¼ cup whole-wheat
   bread crumbs

½ teaspoon dried
   oregano

½ teaspoon dried basil

¼ teaspoon freshly
   ground black pepper

1 cup shredded low-fat
   mozzarella cheese,
   divided

1 Preheat the oven to 350°F.

2 Cut off the ends of the zucchini, and halve them lengthwise.

3 Cut a thin edge off the rounded side of each zucchini half to allow them to lie flat. Scoop out the pulp, leaving ¼-inch-wide shells. Set the pulp aside.

4 Place the boats in a dish that's both microwave- and oven-safe, and add about ¼ cup of water to the bottom of the dish. Cover with a lid or plastic wrap, and microwave on high for 3 minutes, or until the boats are crisp-tender. Drain the liquid from the dish and set the dish aside.

5 Spray a large skillet with cooking spray, and place it over medium heat. Cook the ground beef and onion until the meat is no longer pink and the onion is soft, about 7 minutes. Drain any grease from the skillet and set the skillet aside.

6 In a large bowl, mix together the zucchini pulp, egg, mushrooms, diced tomato, tomato sauce, bread crumbs, oregano, basil, pepper, ½ cup of cheese, and the ground beef and onion mixture.

7 Spoon about ¼ cup of the mixture into each zucchini boat.

8 Sprinkle the tops with the remaining ½ cup of cheese.

9 Bake, uncovered, for 20 minutes, or until the cheese is melted and lightly brown, and serve.

Post-op tip: *Many patients struggle with constipation after bariatric surgery. There can be many reasons for a decrease in the frequency of bowel movements, but for one, most people have decreased fiber intake. A lot of patients have concerns about following a low-carb diet because they feel that grains are the only source of fiber. The good news is that vegetables are just as good a source of fiber, if not better, as whole grains. Focus on getting plenty of veggies in your diet to help keep your gastrointestinal system regular.*

Per Serving (1 zucchini boat): Calories: 162 Total fat: 6g
Sodium: 304mg Total carbs: 11g Sugar: 5g Fiber: 2g Protein: 16g

Post-Op Servings

  ¼ to ½ zucchini boat **G** 1 zucchini boat

Beef and Barley Soup

SERVES 8 / PREP: 15 MINUTES / COOK: 40 MINUTES / TOTAL 55 MINUTES

This classic soup is rich in tender beef that melts in your mouth, and nutty barley, which is an excellent source of soluble fiber and B vitamins important for energy function. No need to serve this soup as a precursor to the main course—it is filling enough for your entire meal.

2 teaspoons extra-virgin olive oil

1½ pounds sirloin steak, cut into 1-inch pieces

1 medium onion, chopped

1 celery stalk, chopped

2 large carrots, chopped

1 medium parsnip, peeled and chopped

1 (6-ounce) can tomato paste

1 tablespoon dried thyme

2 teaspoons Worcestershire sauce

2 teaspoons red wine vinegar

¾ cup quick-cook barley

2 cups beef broth

2 cups water

¼ cup chopped fresh flat-leaf parsley

1 In a large stockpot or Dutch oven over medium heat, heat the olive oil. Add the sirloin pieces, and brown them on all sides, about 5 minutes. Remove the beef from the pot and set aside.

2 Add the onion, celery, carrots, and parsnip to the pot. Cook until tender, about 5 minutes.

3 Mix in the tomato paste, thyme, Worcestershire sauce, and red wine vinegar.

4 Add the beef and barley to the pot, and stir until well coated.

5 Add the broth and water.

6 Bring the soup to a simmer, reduce the heat to low, and cover and cook for 30 minutes, or until the barley is soft and the beef is cooked thoroughly.

7 Serve with the fresh parsley sprinkled on top.

Per Serving (1 cup): Calories: 289 Total fat: 13g Sodium: 288mg
Total carbs: 23g Sugar: 5g Fiber: 5g Protein: 20g

Post-Op Servings

G 1 cup

Beef and Broccoli

SERVES 6 / PREP: 15 MINUTES / COOK: 25 MINUTES / TOTAL: 40 MINUTES

No need for Chinese takeout when you can make tasty beef and broccoli at home. This dish is packed with salty-sweet flavor and plenty of mixed vegetables to get in those essential antioxidants. This reheats well, so it's even better for lunch the next day!

¾ cup beef broth

3 tablespoons apple
cider vinegar

3 tablespoons low-sodium
soy sauce or Bragg
Liquid Aminos

2 tablespoons
brown sugar

1 tablespoon cornstarch

2 teaspoons
ground ginger

¼ teaspoon red
pepper flakes

1 teaspoon sesame oil

2 teaspoons minced garlic

1 pound flank steak, cut
into ¾-inch strips

1 cup broccoli florets

1 red bell pepper, cut into
thin strips

2 bok choy stalks, sliced

1 (8-ounce) can water
chestnuts, drained

Post-Op Servings

G 1 cup

1 In a small bowl, mix together the broth, apple cider vinegar, soy sauce, brown sugar, cornstarch, ginger, and red pepper flakes. Stir until the sugar dissolves. Set aside.

2 In a large skillet over medium heat, heat the sesame oil. Add the garlic, and sauté until fragrant, about 30 seconds. Add the steak, and cook for 2 to 3 minutes on each side. Transfer the steak to a bowl and set aside.

3 With the skillet still over medium heat, add the broccoli and red bell pepper, and sauté for 2 to 3 minutes, stirring constantly.

4 Add the bok choy and water chestnuts, and stir constantly until the bok choy begins to wilt, 3 to 5 minutes.

5 Add the beef and sauce to the skillet. Stir constantly until the sauce thickens, the vegetables are tender, and the beef is cooked through (no longer pink inside), 7 to 10 minutes more, and serve.

Post-op tip: *Beef is not always tolerated after surgery, since it's a very dense meat and difficult mechanically to digest. Swap the beef for chicken or shrimp in this recipe, and you will still have a delicious, protein-rich meal.*

Per Serving (1 cup): Calories: 187 Total fat: 5g Sodium: 461mg
Total carbs: 13g Sugar: 5g Fiber: 2g Protein: 19g

Slow-Cooked Philly Cheesesteak Sandwiches

MAKES 6 SANDWICHES
PREP: 15 MINUTES / COOK: 7 HOURS, 10 MINUTES / TOTAL: 7 HOURS, 25 MINUTES

Here is a fantastic recipe for a slow-cooked beef with typical Philly cheesesteak toppings, but with a healthy twist. The slow-cooked beef is tender and flavorful and a good option if you are starting to experiment with eating more red meat. While doughy bread products are not well tolerated after weight-loss surgery and should be avoided to help keep carbohydrate counts down, most people find that eventually they can tolerate them—but the thinner the better (no large deli rolls).

1½ pounds beef
    chuck roast
½ teaspoon freshly
    ground black pepper
½ teaspoon ground
    marjoram
2 teaspoons extra-virgin
    olive oil
1 large onion, sliced

1 red bell pepper, cut into
    thin strips
1 yellow bell pepper, cut
    into thin strips
8 ounces (2½ cups) sliced
    mini portabella
    mushrooms
½ cup dry red
    cooking wine

1 tablespoon
    Worcestershire sauce
½ cup canned
    tomato sauce
6 sprouted-grain hot
    dog buns, such as
    Angelic Bakehouse, or
    sandwich thins
½ cup shredded
    provolone cheese

1 Sprinkle the pepper and marjoram over the beef.

2 In a large skillet over medium heat, heat the olive oil. Add the beef and sear on both sides, about 3 minutes per side. Transfer the beef to a slow cooker.

3 Add the onion and red and yellow bell peppers to the skillet, and cook for 2 to 3 minutes, until they begin to soften. Add the mushrooms, and cook for 1 minute more.

4 Add the cooking wine and Worcestershire sauce, and bring to a boil. Remove the skillet from the heat.

5 Pour the vegetables and sauce mixture over the roast. Cover the slow cooker, and cook on low for 7 hours until meat is tender and cooked through.

6 Turn off the slow cooker and carefully transfer the roast to a cutting board. Cut the roast into thin slices.

7 Add the tomato sauce to the slow cooker, and mix until well combined.

8 Toast the buns.

9 Layer half of each bun with the beef and top with the vegetables in the tomato sauce. Sprinkle each with the provolone cheese, top with the other half of the bun, and serve.

Per Serving (1 sandwich): Calories: 306 Total fat: 10g Sodium: 386mg Total carbs: 24g Sugar: 2g Fiber: 1g Protein: 30g

Post-Op Servings

G 1 sandwich

Mom's Sloppy Joes

SERVES 8 / PREP: 10 MINUTES / COOK: 30 MINUTES / TOTAL: 40 MINUTES

Revisit your childhood and enjoy this American classic made with wholesome ingredients, more flavors, and less salt than the premade canned versions. This recipe takes me back to memories of quick weeknight meals when my mother was trying to feed four kids in a hurry and on a budget—plus serve us something we actually liked!

Nonstick cooking spray

1½ pounds supreme lean ground beef

1 cup chopped onion

1 cup chopped celery

1 (8-ounce) can tomato sauce

⅓ cup catsup (without high-fructose corn syrup)

2 tablespoons white vinegar

2 tablespoons Worcestershire sauce

2 tablespoons Dijon mustard

1 tablespoon brown sugar

8 100 percent whole-grain thin sandwich rolls, such as Thomas' sandwich thins (optional)

Post-Op Servings

Ⓖ ¾ cup sloppy joe

1 Spray a large skillet with cooking spray, and place it over medium heat. Add the beef and cook until it is no longer pink, about 10 minutes. Drain off any grease.

2 Mix in the onion and celery, and cook for 2 to 3 minutes.

3 Stir in the tomato sauce, catsup, vinegar, Worcestershire sauce, mustard, and brown sugar. Bring the liquid to a simmer, and reduce the heat to low. Cook for 15 minutes, or until the sauce has thickened.

4 Toast the sandwich rolls (if using), spoon about ¾ cup of sloppy joe onto each roll or plate, and serve.

Serving Tip: *With so much flavor, this recipe can be eaten without the bun to keep the carbohydrates down. Otherwise, start by trying these sloppy joes served open faced on half of a toasted thin roll.*

Per Serving (¾ cup): Calories: 269 Total fat: 5g Sodium: 656mg
Total carbs: 32g Sugar: 6g Fiber: 6g Protein: 24g

Low-Carb Cheeseburger Casserole

SERVES 12 / PREP: 10 MINUTES / COOK: 1 HOUR / TOTAL: 1 HOUR, 10 MINUTES

Nothing like a cheeseburger and fries to satisfy you after a hard day of work and to fill the void in an empty stomach—or at least that used to be the case. Just because you can't have the grease and fried food after weight-loss surgery doesn't mean you can't have something that is just as cheesy and beefy, and still has potatoes. Craving curbed.

Nonstick cooking spray

2 pounds supreme lean
    ground beef

1 large onion, minced

2 teaspoons minced garlic

8 small red potatoes,
    washed, imperfections
    cut out, and cut into
    ¼-inch slices

2 eggs

1 (6-ounce) can
    tomato paste

1 cup low-fat milk

¼ teaspoon freshly
    ground black pepper

2 cups shredded
    Cheddar cheese

Post-Op Servings

(G) ¾ cup

1 Preheat the oven to 350°F.

2 Spray a large skillet with cooking spray, and place it over medium heat. Add the ground beef, onion, and garlic, and sauté for about 10 minutes, or until the beef is no longer pink and the onion is tender. Drain off the excess grease and set aside.

3 Coat a 9-by-13-inch casserole dish with cooking spray. Layer the potato slices on the bottom of the dish.

4 In a medium bowl, whisk together the eggs, tomato paste, milk, and pepper until well combined, 2 to 3 minutes.

5 Layer the beef and onion on top of the potatoes, and top this with the egg mixture. Sprinkle the Cheddar cheese evenly over the top of the casserole. Cover the casserole with aluminum foil.

6 Bake for 35 minutes. Remove the foil and bake for 10 minutes more, or until the potatoes are tender and the cheese begins to brown, and serve.

Per Serving (¾ cup) Calories: 244: Total fat: 12g Sodium: 207mg
Total carbs: 11g Sugar: 3g Fiber: 1g Protein: 23g

Slow Cooker Asian Pork Tenderloin

SERVES 8 / PREP: 10 MINUTES, PLUS 20 MINUTES TO MARINATE / COOK: 6 HOURS / TOTAL: 6 HOURS, 30 MINUTES

Pork tenderloin is a lean cut of meat loaded with protein and low in artery-clogging saturated fat. Toss this tenderloin in your slow cooker in the morning and have a tasty hot meal when you return home. Serve this melt-in-your-mouth pork, which has ginger-inspired seasonings, with Asian Cucumber Salad (page 67) on the side. This is an amazing make-ahead freezer meal, too. Follow steps 1 and 2, and then freeze the ingredients in the zip-top bag. Simply thaw for 1 to 2 days in the refrigerator before you plan to make it, and then follow steps 4 and 5 for a delicious dinner.

⅓ cup light soy sauce or Bragg Liquid Aminos

¼ cup brown sugar

2 tablespoons Worcestershire sauce

2 tablespoons freshly squeezed lemon juice

2 tablespoons rice vinegar

1 tablespoon dry mustard

1 tablespoon ground ginger

1½ teaspoons freshly ground black pepper

4 garlic cloves, minced

2 pounds pork tenderloin

Post-Op Servings

Ⓖ 4 ounces

1 In a gallon-size zip-top bag, combine the soy sauce, brown sugar, Worcestershire sauce, lemon juice, rice vinegar, dry mustard, ginger, pepper, and garlic.

2 Add the pork to the bag, seal it, and massage the marinade all over the pork.

3 Refrigerate for at least 20 minutes or, ideally, overnight.

4 Put the pork and marinade in a slow cooker, cover, and cook on low for 4 to 6 hours. Alternatively, bake it for 30 to 40 minutes in a preheated 375°F oven, or until it reaches a minimum internal temperature of 145° F.

5 The pork will be tender and nearly falling apart when it is done.

6 Serve immediately.

Per Serving (4 ounces): Calories: 256 Total Fat: 9g Sodium: 658mg Total carbs: 9g Sugar: 8g Fiber: 0g Total Protein: 34g

Creamy Ranch Pork Chops

SERVES 8 / PREP: 10 MINUTES / COOK: 6 HOURS / TOTAL: 6 HOURS, 10 MINUTES

This classic comfort food recipe tastes better with all-homemade ingredients. You can put this together the night before in the slow cooker, refrigerate the crock, and turn on the slow cooker just before leaving the house in the morning. Knowing there's a delicious hot meal waiting when you get home from work makes the hours go by all the faster. Pork, which can often be a dense meat, turns tender in this recipe and falls apart when served. You can eat these pork chops served with vegetables to keep carbs in check, or serve over potatoes.

4 (8-ounce) bone-in pork chops, either top loin or center loin cuts

1 recipe Homemade Condensed Cream of Mushroom Soup (page 170)

1 cup low-fat milk

1 cup chicken broth

2 tablespoons Ranch Seasoning (page 173)

Post-Op Servings

G ½ pork chop

1 Place the pork chops in a slow cooker, and pour the mushroom soup, milk, and broth over them.

2 Mix in the ranch seasoning to coat well.

3 Cover the slow cooker, and cook on low for 6 hours. The pork chops are done when they're tender and nearly falling off the bone.

4 Serve immediately.

Did you know? *Pork (and all meats, eggs, and dairy) is an excellent source of vitamin B_{12}, which is important for preventing anemia and crucial for nerve function. Due to changes in the absorption of vitamin B_{12} and a risk of its deficiency after bariatric surgery, many patients need a B_{12} supplement in the form of a pill or injection.*

Per Serving (½ pork chop): Calories: 180 Total fat: 6g Sodium: 700mg
Total carbs: 14g Sugar: 3g Fiber: 1g Protein: 13g

Naked Pulled Pork

SERVES 8 / PREP: 20 MINUTES / COOK: 6 HOURS / TOTAL 6 HOURS, 20 MINUTES

Try this slow-cooked Texas-style pulled pork, which takes an otherwise tough cut of meat and makes it oh so tender. Top this with healthy creamy coleslaw to balance out the zesty seasonings in the pork.

For the pork

2 (15-ounce) cans tomato sauce

3 tablespoons onion powder

2 tablespoons garlic powder

1 tablespoon ground cumin

1 tablespoon brown sugar

2 teaspoons Chili Powder (page 175)

1 teaspoon ground cinnamon

½ teaspoon ground cayenne pepper

2 pounds pork shoulder, trimmed of excess fat

1 medium onion, diced

For the creamy coleslaw

⅔ cup low-fat plain Greek yogurt

2 tablespoons apple cider vinegar

1 tablespoon freshly squeezed lemon juice

1 teaspoon honey

1 teaspoon Dijon mustard

1 teaspoon onion powder

1 teaspoon celery seed

2 cups shredded green cabbage

2 cups shredded red cabbage

1 cup shredded carrots

½ cup chopped scallions

TO PREPARE THE PORK

1 In a small bowl, mix together the tomato sauce, onion powder, garlic powder, cumin, brown sugar, chili powder, cinnamon, and cayenne pepper.

2 Place the pork shoulder and onion in the slow cooker, and pour the sauce over them.

3 Cover the slow cooker, and cook on low for 6 hours.

4 The finished pork should shred easily. Use two forks to shred the pork in the slow cooker. If there is any additional sauce, allow the pork to cook on low for 20 minutes more to absorb the remaining liquid.

TO PREPARE THE CREAMY COLESLAW

1 In a small bowl, mix together the yogurt, vinegar, lemon juice, honey, mustard, onion powder, and celery seed.

2 In a large bowl, combine the green and red cabbage, carrots, and scallions. Pour the dressing over the vegetables, and toss to coat well. For best results, refrigerate the coleslaw overnight.

3 Serve the pork topped with the coleslaw.

Per Serving (½ cup pork with ½ cup coleslaw): Calories: 260
Total fat: 11g Sodium: 705mg Total carbs: 20g Sugar: 10g Fiber: 5g
Protein: 20g

Post-Op Servings

(G) ½ cup pork with ½ cup coleslaw

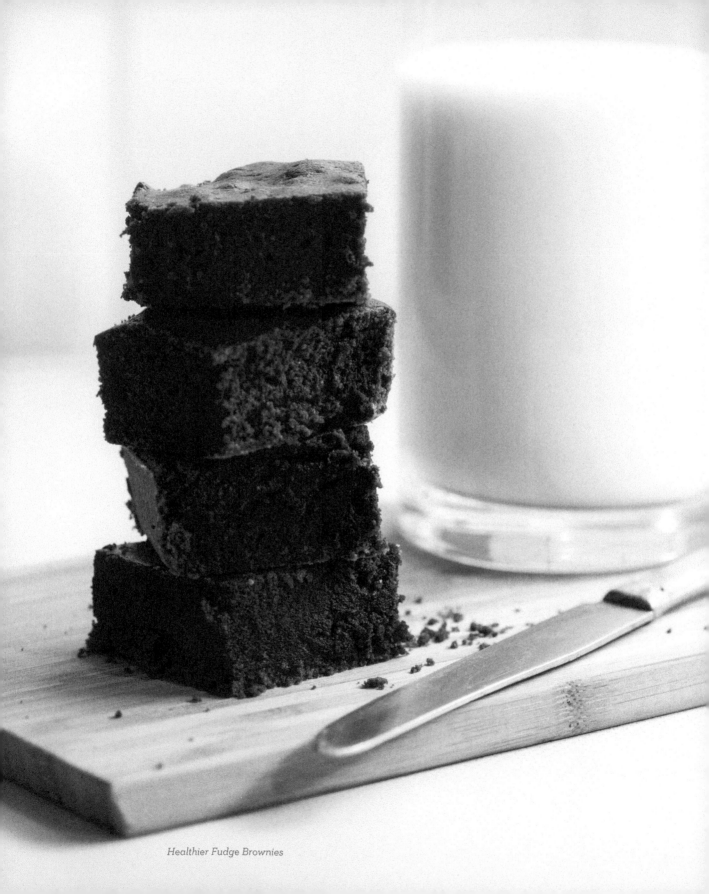

Healthier Fudge Brownies

CHAPTER NINE

Drinks and Desserts

Fruit-Infused Waters

MAKES ABOUT 2 CUPS / PREP: 10 MINUTES / TOTAL: 10 MINUTES

Although artificial sweeteners are safe to have after surgery, there is something to be said about trying to drink clean beverages free of both sugar and any artificial sugar substitutes. For some people, drinking excessive amounts of sugary beverages may cause cravings for other sugary foods. Infused waters are a tasty option for having a flavorful drink without sugar or a substitute. And the options are endless when choosing what to put in your fruit-infused water—be creative and experiment with a variety of herbs and spices. Increasing the flavor in your water may help you reach your fluid goals for the day.

Infuser options:

3 to 5 cucumber slices, 2 lime wedges, and 4 fresh mint leaves

4 sliced strawberries and ¼ jalapeño pepper

4 fresh basil leaves and ¼ cup cubed watermelon

1 fresh rosemary sprig, stemmed, and ¼ cup grapefruit wedges

2 or 3 blackberries, ⅛ cup blueberries, and 2 orange wedges

2 lemon wedges, 2 lime wedges, and 2 orange wedges

2 cucumber slices, ½ fresh lavender sprig, stemmed, 3 fresh mint leaves, and 2 lemon wedges

¼ apple, sliced, and 1 teaspoon ground cinnamon or 1 cinnamon stick

1 Mix any of the preceding combinations with at least 2 cups of water.

2 If using herbs, use a wooden spoon or muddler to muddle them with the fruit to help bring out their flavors.

3 Consider using an infuser bottle or pitcher to help separate seeds and herbs so they don't mix into the drinkable portion of the water.

Per Serving (1 cup): Calories: 0 Total fat: 0g Sodium: 0mg
Total carbs: 0g Sugar: 0g Fiber: 0g Protein: 0g

Post-Op Servings

P S G

1 to 8 cups a day

Refreshing Mint Lemonade

MAKES 4 CUPS / PREP: 10 MINUTES / TOTAL: 10 MINUTES

All sugary beverages should become a thing of the past after bariatric surgery, but no need to feel obligated to stick to plain water all the time. Try this refreshing twist on lemonade to give some variety to your beverages. It's made with all-natural plant-based stevia, which provides no calories and no carbohydrates but is sweeter than sugar.

Juice of 2 lemons

2 fresh mint sprigs

½ teaspoon stevia powder

4 cups water

Ice

1 In a small pitcher, use a wooden spoon or muddler to muddle together the lemon juice, mint leaves, and stevia to help bring out the oils in the mint.

2 Fill the pitcher with the water and ice, and serve.

Per Serving (1 cup): Calories: 5 Total fat: 0g Sodium: 0mg
Total carbs: 1g Sugar: 0g Fiber: 0g Protein: 0g

Post-Op Servings

P S G

1 to 4 cups a day

Healthier Fudge Brownies

MAKES 16 BROWNIES / PREP: 10 MINUTES / COOK: 30 MINUTES / TOTAL: 40 MINUTES

These brownies have a secret ingredient, one that anyone who tastes them (other than you, their baker) will never, ever guess. That ingredient is beans— yes, black beans. While the beans don't affect the brownie flavor at all, they help create an irresistible fudgy texture. I'm not lying when I say they're tastier than the box version, plus being lower in sugar and fat. Bring these treats to your next potluck, party, or birthday celebration as a treat you can safely enjoy.

Nonstick cooking spray

1 (14.5-ounce) can
    black beans, drained
    and rinsed

3 eggs

3 tablespoons canola oil

¼ cup unsweetened
    cocoa powder

1 teaspoon vanilla extract

⅓ cup granulated sugar

1 teaspoon instant coffee
    (optional)

½ cup dark chocolate chips

1 Preheat the oven to 350°F. Coat an 8-by-8-inch square baking dish with cooking spray.

2 In a blender, blend to combine the black beans, eggs, canola oil, cocoa powder, vanilla, sugar, and coffee (if using) until smooth and lump free.

3 Pour the mixture into the baking dish, and sprinkle the chocolate chips on top.

4 Bake until the top is dry and the edges start to pull away from the sides of the pan, about 30 minutes.

5 Cut into 16 brownies and serve.

Per Serving (1 brownie) : Calories: 124 Total fat: 6g Sodium: 18mg
Total carbs: 16g Sugar: 7g Fiber: 5g Protein: 4g

Post-Op Servings

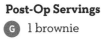 1 brownie

Creamy Pumpkin Mousse

SERVES 10 / PREP: 15 MINUTES / TOTAL: 15 MINUTES

Nothing screams fall like pumpkin. With its creamy, silky texture, it's the perfect ingredient for a tasty dessert. This mousse has a cheesecake-like texture that will certainly satisfy your sweet tooth. Use Neufchâtel cream cheese instead of regular cream cheese to save a few calories and some saturated fat. Don't forget to sprinkle the cinnamon on top to finish off this scrumptious dessert that's so good, you'll serve it all year-round.

2 (8-ounce) packages Neufchâtel cream cheese, at room temperature

1 (15-ounce) can pumpkin puree

2 cups low-fat milk

2 teaspoons pumpkin pie spice

2 teaspoons liquid stevia

1 teaspoon vanilla extract

1 teaspoon ground cinnamon

Post-Op Servings

Ⓖ ⅔ cup

1 In a medium bowl, use a hand mixer to blend the cream cheese and pumpkin puree until smooth and well combined.

2 Add the milk, pumpkin pie spice, stevia, and vanilla, and continue to blend for 5 minutes more, or until the mixture is light and airy.

3 Place about ⅔ cup of mousse in each serving glass, and sprinkle the top with the cinnamon. Refrigerate until ready to serve.

Did you know? *Pumpkin is an excellent source of beta-carotene, which is an antioxidant shown to attack damaging free radicals in the body and protect against cancer and heart disease. Other sources of beta-carotene include carrots and squash.*

Per Serving (⅔ cup) : Calories: 151 Total fat: 10g Sodium: 177mg Total carbs: 7g Fiber: 0g Sugar: 5g Protein: 6g

Vanilla Cheesecake Parfaits

MAKES 4 PARFAITS / PREP: 30 MINUTES / TOTAL: 30 MINUTES

Bite into a freshly picked strawberry, blueberry, or blackberry at the height of their harvest, and you experience an explosion of sweet and tart in your mouth all at once. These berries are the perfect accompaniment to a creamy cheesecake filling. This recipe uses tofu as a hidden ingredient to give the creamy texture without adding extra fat and calories. To serve, make sure to use clear glasses—I like to use a stemless wine glass or water glass—so you can admire the beauty in the berries!

¾ cup low-fat plain Greek yogurt

3 ounces silken tofu (about one-fifth of a 16-ounce package)

¾ teaspoon powdered stevia extract

2 teaspoons vanilla extract

1 cup blackberries, cut into thirds

1 cup strawberries, stemmed and quartered

1 cup blueberries

4 fresh mint leaves

Post-Op Servings

Ⓖ 1 parfait

1 In a large mixing bowl, use a hand mixer on medium-high speed to beat the yogurt, tofu, stevia, and vanilla until creamy, fluffy, and completely smooth.

2 Prepare 4 small (8-ounce) glasses to layer the parfaits in.

3 To create the parfaits, layer the blackberries in the bottom of the glasses, layer a dollop of the yogurt mixture on top of them, layer the strawberries next, and layer another dollop of the yogurt mixture. Layer the blueberries, and end with a final dollop of yogurt mixture. Garnish each glass with a mint leaf.

4 Refrigerate until ready to serve.

Did you know? *Berries are an excellent source of vitamins and antioxidants and are a top superfood to include in your diet. Each color represents different phytochemicals that can have beneficial effects in the body. Switch this recipe up and include your favorite fresh berries— raspberries (red or white), black currants, tart cranberries— whatever is available to you and in season.*

Per Serving (1 parfait): Calories: 103 Total fat: 2g Sodium: 28mg Total carbs: 15g Sugar: 9g Fiber: 4g Protein: 6g

Lemon Bars

MAKES 24 BARS / PREP: 10 MINUTES / COOK: 35 MINUTES / TOTAL: 45 MINUTES

A tangy, tart lemon dessert makes for a delightful and refreshing treat. You don't have to worry about going overboard with your sugar intake while eating these lemon bars. They're made with stevia extract to keep calories and carbohydrates at a minimum. While coconut oil should be restricted in the diet because it's a saturated fat, it's an excellent alternative, when used in moderation, to butter and lard. Here it makes a crispy crust possible.

For the crust

Nonstick cooking spray

1 cup whole-wheat
    pastry flour

¼ cup stevia baking blend

¼ cup coconut oil

For the lemon filling

4 eggs

2 egg yolks

½ cup stevia baking blend

Juice of 4 lemons

2 tablespoons coconut oil

Post-Op Servings

Ⓖ 1 bar

TO PREPARE THE CRUST

1 Preheat the oven to 350°F. Spray a 9-by-13-inch baking pan with cooking spray.

2 In a medium mixing bowl, use a hand blender on medium-high speed to blend the flour, stevia, and coconut oil until the mixture becomes coarse.

3 Transfer the mixture to the baking pan, pressing it into the bottom to form a thin, even layer.

4 Bake for 20 minutes, or until the crust begins to turn a golden brown. Remove the pan from the oven but do not turn off the oven. Allow the crust to cool for about 5 minutes before adding the filling.

TO PREPARE THE LEMON FILLING

1 While the crust bakes, in a small saucepan, whisk the eggs, egg yolks, and stevia until well combined. Place the pan over medium heat, and stir in the lemon juice and coconut oil. Cook the filling for 5 minutes, stirring frequently, until the mixture thickens.

2 Pour the filling over the baked crust, and bake for an additional 14 to 15 minutes. It is done when the edges begin to brown and the filling has solidified.

3 Cool completely, cut into 24 bars, and serve.

Per Serving (1 bar): Calories: 55 Total fat: 4g Sodium: 13mg
Total carbs: 4g Sugar: 7g Fiber: 1g Protein: 2g

Creamy Chocolate Fruit Dip

MAKES 9 SERVINGS
PREP: 10 MINUTES, PLUS 30 MINUTES TO CHILL / TOTAL: 40 MINUTES

We all know we are supposed to fill up on fruits and vegetables throughout the day, but sometimes it's uninspiring just to eat them plain. I often hear this complaint from parents who struggle to get their children to eat fruits and vegetables. Try this fruit dip to jazz up plain fruit and help you eat fruit more often. As an added bonus, you will even get some protein.

1½ cups low-fat plain Greek yogurt

½ cup creamy natural peanut butter

2 tablespoons honey

2 tablespoons unsweetened cocoa powder

1 teaspoon vanilla extract

Post-Op Servings

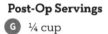 ¼ cup

1 In a medium mixing bowl, use a hand mixer on low speed to beat together the yogurt, peanut butter, honey, cocoa powder, and vanilla just until smooth and well combined.

2 Cover and refrigerate overnight, or for at least 30 minutes prior to serving, to meld the flavors.

3 Keep chilled while serving.

Serving tip: *Serve with fresh fruit such as apple, pear, or banana slices. Some patients may tolerate fresh fruit better post-op without the skin, especially when transitioning to fresh fruits and vegetables for the first time.*

Per Serving (¼ cup) : Calories: 120 Total fat: 7g Sodium: 53mg
Total carbs: 10g Fiber: 1g Sugar: 7g Protein: 6g

Heart-Healthy Peanut Butter–Chocolate Chip Cookies

MAKES 4 DOZEN COOKIES
PREP: 15 MINUTES / COOK: 10 MINUTES / TOTAL: 25 MINUTES

Chocolate chip cookies are a familiar part of our life and culture—whether as a snack after school dipped in milk, upon check-in at your hotel while on vacation, or at Grandma's house when you go to visit. It's hard to imagine life without this tasty dessert. Here is a healthier twist on chocolate chip cookies—packed with creamy peanut butter and heart-healthy oil.

½ cup creamy natural peanut butter

⅓ cup canola oil

¼ cup granulated sugar

¼ cup packed brown sugar

1 teaspoon vanilla extract

2 large eggs

1¼ cups old-fashioned rolled oats

1 cup whole-wheat pastry flour

2 tablespoons ground flaxseed

1 teaspoon baking soda

⅔ cup dark chocolate chips (60 percent cacao or higher)

1 Preheat the oven to 350°F.

2 In a large mixing bowl, use a hand mixer to beat the peanut butter, canola oil, granulated and brown sugars, and vanilla until creamy and smooth.

3 Beat in the eggs one at a time.

4 In a small bowl, mix together the oats, flour, flaxseed, and baking soda.

5 Gradually beat the dry ingredients into the peanut butter mixture.

6 Stir in the chocolate chips.

7 Drop teaspoons of dough onto an ungreased baking sheet about 2 inches apart.

8 Bake for about 9 minutes, or until the edges begin to brown.

9 Let the cookies cool on the baking sheet for about 1 minute, and then with a spatula transfer them to a cooling rack to cool completely before serving.

Did you know? *Flaxseed is an excellent source of fiber, omega-3 fatty acid, and alpha-linolenic acid (ALA). Flaxseed has been shown to help lower blood pressure, among many other health benefits. Mix a tablespoon into your protein shake, spaghetti sauce, meatloaf, or any baked goods to sneak it in!*

Per Serving (2 cookies): Calories: 164 Total fat: 10g Sodium: 75mg Total carbs: 17g Sugar: 8g Fiber: 2g Protein: 3g

Post-Op Servings

(G) 2 cookies

Low-Carb Chocolate Mousse

SERVES 4
PREP: 10 MINUTES, PLUS AT LEAST 2 HOURS TO CHILL / TOTAL: 2 HOURS, 10 MINUTES

This creamy, rich chocolate mousse will transport you to heaven. You truly can still enjoy dessert without all the added sugar since this recipe requires only stevia powder to sweeten it. The chia seeds are used to help the mixture thicken naturally without traditional ingredients like heavy whipped cream. Topping the finished mousse with fresh raspberries adds a pop of rich color and a tangy finish.

1 cup low-fat
  ricotta cheese
1 cup low-fat milk
1 tablespoon
  unsweetened
  cocoa powder
1 tablespoon chia seeds
2 teaspoons stevia powder
½ teaspoon vanilla extract
1 cup raspberries

Post-Op Servings
Ⓖ ½ cup

1 In a blender, blend on medium speed to combine the ricotta, milk, cocoa powder, chia seeds, stevia, and vanilla until well blended and very smooth.

2 Divide the mousse evenly among 4 small serving glasses.

3 Refrigerate for at least 2 hours to thicken, or overnight for best results.

4 Top each glass with ¼ cup of fresh raspberries and serve.

Did you know? *Chia seeds are an excellent source of fiber and omega-3 fats. One tablespoon packs a whopping 4.5 grams of fiber! Try them tossed into your yogurt in the morning to add in some extra nutrients and help meet your fiber goal for the day.*

Per Serving (½ cup) : Calories: 113 Total fat: 3g Sodium: 102mg
Total carbs: 13g Sugar: 8g Fiber: 7g Protein: 9g

Raspberry Frozen Yogurt

MAKES 4 CUPS / PREP: 10 MINUTES / TOTAL: 10 MINUTES

Ice cream and frozen yogurt are missed by many patients after weight-loss surgery. There's nothing like something cool and fruity on a hot summer day. Fortunately, this frozen yogurt is sweet and tart and will satisfy your urge for ice cream. That it takes just four ingredients and can be made in less than 10 minutes means you can enjoy this dessert all summer long.

4 cups frozen raspberries

½ cup low-fat plain Greek yogurt

2 tablespoons freshly squeezed lemon juice

2 teaspoons liquid stevia

Post-Op Servings

(G) 1 cup

1 In a blender or food processor, blend to combine the raspberries, yogurt, lemon juice, and stevia until smooth, about 5 minutes.

2 Serve immediately, or freeze in an airtight container and use within 3 weeks.

Serving tip: *Substitute any of your favorite fruits to keep variety in this frozen yogurt recipe. Try frozen strawberries, peaches, or mangos!*

Per Serving (1 cup): Calories: 114 Total fat: 2g Sodium: 18mg Total carbs: 19g Sugar: 7g Fiber: 9g Protein: 5g

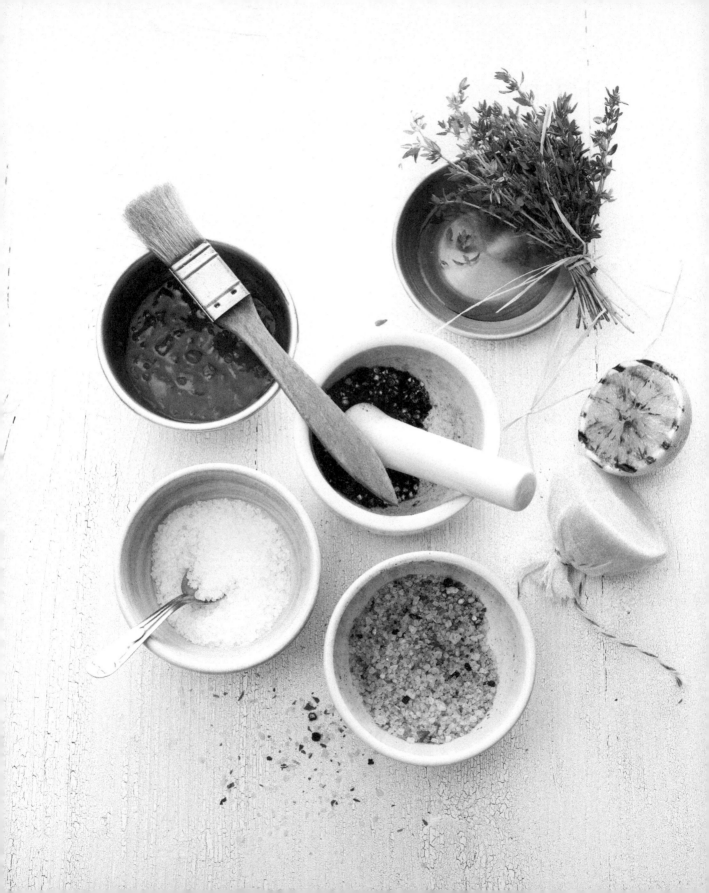

CHAPTER TEN

Dressings, Sauces, and Seasonings

Avocado-Lime Dressing

MAKES 2 CUPS / PREP: 10 MINUTES / TOTAL: 10 MINUTES

This rich and creamy dressing is perfect to top a fresh salad, jazz up plain chicken, add flavor to tacos or beef, or transform a boring turkey wrap into something extra tasty. Portion this dressing into small containers to take with you for meals on the go, or keep sealed tightly in the refrigerator for about a week.

½ cup water

1 very ripe avocado

¼ cup low-fat plain
  Greek yogurt

¼ cup chopped fresh
  cilantro

3 tablespoons extra-virgin
  olive oil

Juice of 1 lime (about
  2 tablespoons)

1 teaspoon minced garlic

¼ teaspoon ground
  cayenne pepper

¼ teaspoon freshly
  ground black pepper

Post-Op Servings

P S G

2 tablespoons

In a blender or food processor, puree the water, avocado, yogurt, cilantro, olive oil, lime juice, garlic, cayenne pepper, and black pepper on medium-high speed until the dressing has a creamy texture and there are no chunks.

Ingredient tip: *Here's the fastest way to peel an avocado:*

- *Carefully cut the avocado in half with a sharp knife, rotating around the pit.*
- *Gently twist the two halves to break it apart.*
- *Using the sharp edge of the knife (not the point), stab the pit, and twist the knife to remove the pit. Discard the pit.*
- *Scoop out the avocado flesh with a spoon.*
- *Drizzle lemon or lime juice over leftover avocado to prevent browning, and store it in an airtight container in the refrigerator.*

Per Serving (2 tablespoons): Calories: 50 Total fat: 4g Sodium: 4mg
Total carbs: 2g Sugar: 0g Fiber: 1g Protein: 1g

Low-Fat Caesar Dressing

MAKES 1 CUP / PREP: 10 MINUTES / TOTAL: 10 MINUTES

The days of a Caesar salad with Parmesan cheese are not over just because you had bariatric surgery. Most of the bottled Caesar salad dressings are loaded with fat, but this homemade version is made with Greek yogurt to give the same texture without the extra calories. Don't forget the anchovy fillets—you can find them in the canned section of your grocery store. They are essential for giving this dressing its true Caesar flavor. Once you've pureed the dressing, you won't even know they are there.

½ cup low-fat plain Greek yogurt

½ cup shredded Parmesan cheese

¼ cup freshly squeezed lemon juice

¼ cup low-fat milk

1 tablespoon extra-virgin olive oil

2 anchovy fillets, jarred or canned

2 teaspoons Worcestershire sauce

1 teaspoon minced garlic

1 teaspoon Dijon mustard

1 teaspoon onion powder

½ teaspoon freshly ground black pepper

In a blender or food processor, puree the yogurt, cheese, lemon juice, milk, olive oil, anchovies, Worcestershire sauce, garlic, mustard, onion powder, and pepper on medium-high speed until the dressing is smooth and creamy without any lumps.

Post-op tip: *Want the Caesar salad flavor quick on the pureed diet? Puree 1 to 2 tablespoons dressing with canned chicken for a tasty meal made in less than 5 minutes.*

Per Serving (2 tablespoons): Calories: 48 Total fat: 4g Sodium: 111mg
Total carbs: 2g Sugar: 1g Fiber: 0g Protein: 4g

Post-Op Servings

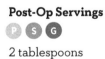

2 tablespoons

Quick Stir-Fry Sauce

MAKES 2 CUPS / PREP: 10 MINUTES / COOK: 5 MINUTES / TOTAL: 15 MINUTES

Many jarred stir-fry sauces are packed with unhealthy high-fructose corn syrup, sodium, and a list of ingredients I cannot even pronounce! Save money and enjoy improved flavor by making your own stir-fry sauce.

½ cup low-sodium
   soy sauce

½ cup chicken or
   vegetable broth

3 tablespoons catsup
   (free from high-fructose
   corn syrup)

2 tablespoons rice vinegar

1 tablespoon sesame oil

1 tablespoon brown sugar

1½ teaspoons honey

1 teaspoon sriracha or
   other hot sauce

¼ teaspoon freshly
   ground black pepper

½ cup cold water

2 tablespoons cornstarch

2 tablespoons extra-virgin
   olive oil

1 tablespoon
   minced garlic

1 teaspoon ground ginger

1 In a medium bowl, stir to combine the soy sauce, broth, catsup, rice vinegar, sesame oil, brown sugar, honey, sriracha, and pepper. Set aside.

2 In a small bowl, mix together the water and cornstarch until there are no lumps. Set aside.

3 In a small saucepan over medium heat, heat the olive oil. Sauté the garlic and ginger just until the oil begins to simmer, 1 to 2 minutes.

4 Whisk in the soy sauce mixture, and bring the liquid to a boil.

5 Slowly whisk in the cornstarch mixture. Cook the sauce for a few minutes more until it has thickened, stirring constantly.

6 Store the sauce in an airtight container in the refrigerator for up to 1 week or freeze for up to 1 month. Reheat the sauce and stir well before using.

Per Serving (¼ cup): Calories: 93 Total fat: 5g Sodium: 846mg
Total carbs: 10g Sugar: 4g Fiber: 0g Protein: 2g

Post-Op Servings

P S G

¼ cup

Seafood Sauce

MAKES 2 CUPS / PREP: 10 MINUTES, PLUS 30 MINUTES TO CHILL / TOTAL: 40 MINUTES

We already know that boiled or baked seafood is one of the lowest-calorie ways to eat protein, plus you get all those brain- and heart-healthy omega-3s. But you don't have to eat it plain. Adding a little seafood sauce, rich with flavor from fresh lemon and horseradish, can take your seafood from boring to a zesty party in your mouth.

1½ cups catsup (free from high-fructose corn syrup)

2 tablespoons grated horseradish

Juice of 1 lemon

1 tablespoon Worcestershire sauce

1 teaspoon Chili Powder (page 175)

¼ teaspoon freshly ground black pepper

Post-Op Servings

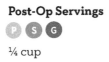

¼ cup

1 In a small bowl, mix to combine the catsup, horseradish, lemon juice, Worcestershire sauce, chili powder, and pepper. Refrigerate, covered, for at least 30 minutes or overnight to let the flavors meld.

2 Serve with shrimp cocktail, oysters, grilled scallops, or other seafood.

Post-op tip: *Use this as a base to enjoy your favorite seafood selections on the pureed diet.*

Per Serving (¼ cup): Calories: 56 Total fat: 0g Sodium: 445mg Total carbs: 14g Sugar: 10g Fiber: 0g Protein: 0g

Homemade Condensed Cream of Mushroom Soup

MAKES 1 (10.75-OUNCE) CAN EQUIVALENT
PREP: 10 MINUTES / COOK: 10 MINUTES / TOTAL: 20 MINUTES

Creamed soups are loaded with fat and calories, and low-fat versions tend to be excessively high in sodium. Try replacing canned condensed cream of mushroom soup with this recipe, which is packed with flavor, whole chunks of real mushrooms, and a creamy texture.

4 teaspoons extra-virgin olive oil, divided

4 ounces mushrooms

2 tablespoons whole-wheat pastry flour

½ cup vegetable or chicken broth

½ cup low-fat milk

½ teaspoon freshly ground black pepper

Post-Op Servings

P S G

⅛ cup used in preparing recipes

1 In a medium skillet over medium heat, heat 1 teaspoon of olive oil. Add the mushrooms, and sauté until tender, about 5 minutes. Remove the skillet and set aside.

2 In a medium saucepan over medium heat, heat the remaining 3 teaspoons of olive oil.

3 Gradually add the flour, and stir constantly until it is blended with the oil and the mixture is smooth. Turn off the heat.

4 Slowly add the broth and milk, whisking constantly until the mixture is smooth.

5 Stir in the mushrooms, and bring the mixture to a boil over medium-high heat. Stir in the pepper, reduce the heat to low, and simmer for 5 minutes.

6 Use as a substitute for 1 (10.75-ounce) can of condensed cream of mushroom soup in recipes.

Did you know? *Mushrooms are a good source of minerals such as zinc, copper, and selenium. Initially after weight-loss surgery, intake of these minerals can be low for many patients. Zinc is essential for proper growth and maintenance of tissue in the body including wound healing.*

Per Serving (⅛ cup): Calories: 39 Total fat: 3g Sodium: 41mg
Total carbs: 3g Sugar: 0g Fiber: 0g Protein: 1g

Creamy Alfredo Sauce

MAKES 4 CUPS / PREP: 5 MINUTES / COOK: 10 MINUTES / TOTAL: 15 MINUTES

If you thought that you could never allow yourself the treat of Alfredo sauce again, I'm happy to introduce you to this recipe. Free of butter and heavy cream, it's entirely bariatric-friendly while also delivering the flavors that make this classic sauce so delicious. It's easy to prepare and is a great topping for fish, seafood, vegetables, or poultry. Try it over spaghetti squash or zucchini noodles (zoodles) instead of pasta for an especially low-carb, tasty meal.

2 teaspoons extra-virgin olive oil

4 teaspoons minced garlic

3 tablespoons whole-wheat pastry flour

1 cup vegetable or chicken broth

2 cups fat-free or 1 percent milk

¼ teaspoon freshly ground black pepper

6 ounces shredded Parmesan cheese

¼ cup chopped fresh parsley, for garnish

1 In a medium pot over medium-high heat, heat the olive oil. Add the garlic, and sauté for 1 minute.

2 Add the flour and mix, stirring constantly, to form a paste, 2 to 3 minutes.

3 Whisk in the broth, and then slowly whisk in the milk. Cook for 2 to 3 minutes more.

4 Season the sauce with the pepper, and stir in the Parmesan cheese just until it is melted. Remove the pot from the heat.

5 Garnish the sauce with the fresh parsley before serving.

Per Serving (¼ cup): Calories: 72 Total fat: 4g Sodium: 229mg
Total carbs: 4g Sugar: 0g Fiber: 0g Protein: 5g

Post-Op Servings

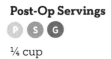

¼ cup

Fresh Salsa

MAKES 2 CUPS / PREP: 15 MINUTES / TOTAL: 15 MINUTES

Salsa is a condiment where you can't go wrong. Loaded with vegetables and seasonings, it's almost always a good choice. The problem is what we use to dip in the salsa! Mix up a batch of this fresh salsa and use it more as a condiment and less as a dip for chips. The flavors from the fresh seasonings surpass any jarred version on store shelves. Serve over eggs, dollop on a Naked Burrito Salad (page 82), or use to garnish grilled chicken or fish.

3 medium tomatoes, diced

⅓ cup chopped green
   bell pepper

¼ cup chopped onion

¼ cup chopped scallions

1 teaspoon apple cider
   vinegar

1 teaspoon freshly
   squeezed lemon juice

1 teaspoon extra-virgin
   olive oil

1 teaspoon minced
   jalapeño pepper

1 teaspoon ground cumin

¼ teaspoon salt

¼ teaspoon ground
   cayenne pepper

¼ cup fresh chopped
   fresh cilantro

In a medium bowl, mix together the tomatoes, bell pepper, onion, scallions, vinegar, lemon juice, olive oil, jalapeño, cumin, salt, cayenne pepper, and cilantro. Enjoy immediately, or refrigerate for up to 3 days.

Per Serving (¼ cup): Calories: 16 Total fat: 0g Sodium: 76mg
Total carbs: 3g Sugar: 2g Fiber: 1g Protein: 1g

Post-Op Servings

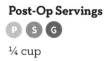

¼ cup

Seasoning Recipes

No need to worry about buying special seasoning mixes for cooking when you can easily make a batch of your own with items already in your pantry. Some seasoning mixes contain added sugars, artificial colorings, fillers, and high amounts of sodium. By making your own using dried herbs without additives, you will have a clean product, and the taste is incredible when freshly mixed together compared to using something that's been sitting on the store shelf for months. Even better, you can make these and keep them in an airtight container in your pantry for up to three months. Now that's easy access. All of these seasonings are 100 percent free of calories, fat, sugar, carbohydrates, and sodium!

Ranch Seasoning

MAKES ¼ CUP / PREP: 5 MINUTES / TOTAL: 5 MINUTES

2 tablespoons
    dried parsley

1½ teaspoons dried dill

1 teaspoon garlic powder

1 teaspoon onion powder

½ teaspoon dried basil

½ teaspoon freshly
    ground black pepper

In a container with an airtight lid, combine the parsley, dill, garlic powder, onion powder, basil, and pepper. Put the lid on, give the container a few shakes, and store it in your pantry until ready to use.

Serving tip: *Add creamy ranch flavor to any dish with this seasoning. Sprinkle it over chicken breast or mix it into low-fat cottage cheese or tuna or chicken salad.*

Taco Seasoning

MAKES ABOUT 2½ TABLESPOONS / PREP: 5 MINUTES / TOTAL: 5 MINUTES

¾ teaspoon garlic powder

½ teaspoon onion powder

¼ teaspoon red
pepper flakes

¾ teaspoon dried
oregano

2 teaspoons ground
paprika

1 teaspoon freshly ground
black pepper

2 teaspoons ground cumin

½ teaspoon ground
cayenne pepper

In a container with an airtight lid, combine the garlic powder, onion powder, red pepper flakes, oregano, paprika, black pepper, cumin, and cayenne pepper. Put the lid on, give the container a few shakes, and store it in your pantry until ready to use.

Post-op tip: *Use this in all your favorite Tex-Mex dishes. Add some variety to your cottage cheese in the pureed diet by mixing in a dash of this seasoning.*

Cajun Seasoning

MAKES 3½ TABLESPOONS / PREP: 5 MINUTES / TOTAL: 5 MINUTES

1½ tablespoons ground
paprika

1½ teaspoons
onion powder

1½ teaspoons
garlic powder

½ teaspoon freshly
ground black pepper

1 teaspoon ground
cayenne pepper

½ teaspoon ground cumin

½ teaspoon dried thyme

½ teaspoon dried
oregano

In a container with an airtight lid, combine the paprika, onion powder, garlic powder, black pepper, cayenne pepper, cumin, thyme, and oregano. Put the lid on, give the container a few shakes, and store it in your pantry until ready to use.

Serving tip: *Use this Cajun seasoning as a coating for chicken or fish. Just sprinkle some on before you bake or panfry. You won't miss the breading, and you won't miss the extra fat or calories.*

Chili Powder

2½ tablespoons ground paprika

2 teaspoons dried oregano

1½ teaspoons ground cumin

1½ teaspoons garlic powder

1½ teaspoons ground cayenne pepper

¾ teaspoon onion powder

¼ teaspoon ground cloves

¼ teaspoon ground allspice

In a container with an airtight lid, combine the paprika, oregano, cumin, garlic powder, cayenne pepper, onion powder, cloves, and allspice. Put the lid on, give the container a few shakes, and store it in your pantry until ready to use.

Serving tip: *Besides flavoring the traditional pot-o-chili, this chili powder can be used to season eggs or ground meat for a change of pace and delicious flavor. Add more cayenne pepper to this recipe if you like the taste extra spicy.*

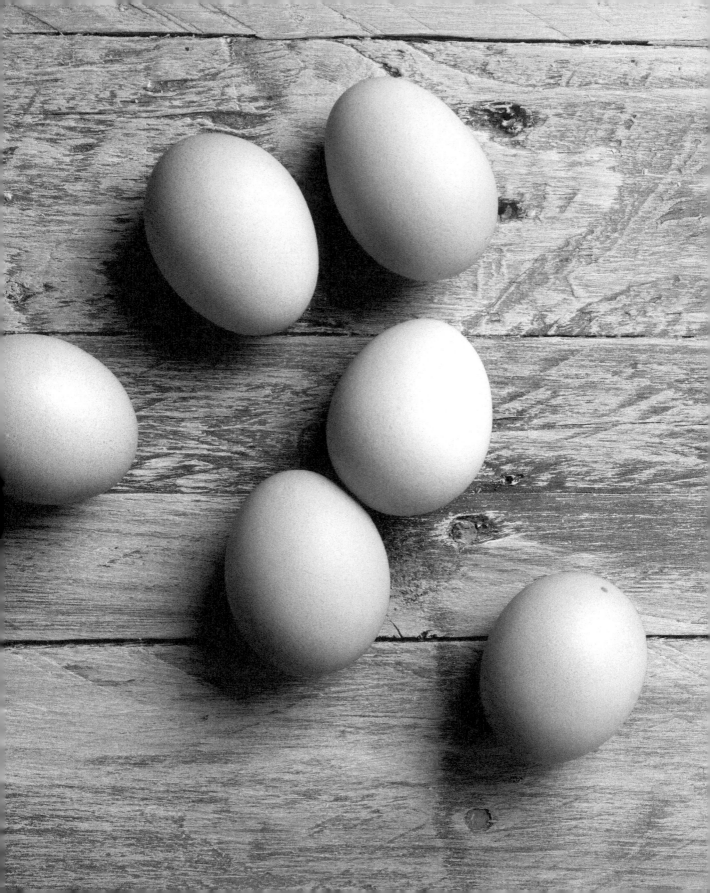

Tips for Eating at Restaurants
or in Others' Homes

Wouldn't it be nice if we could have home-cooked meals every single night with clean, fresh ingredients? Although this is a goal and hopefully something that you have integrated into your lifestyle, there are undoubtedly going to be times when you may eat in a restaurant or in someone else's home. Wait until at least three months after surgery before you venture into dining away from home if at all possible—you will have much better insight about which foods you can tolerate and which ones upset your new pouch.

Here are a few tips to help you follow your weight-loss plan when you are out and about:

▶ **Ask for what you need.** Don't forget, you are paying for the meal and the service when you go out to eat. Ask your server as many questions as needed to make sure you know exactly how your meal is prepared. Let them know you are on a special diet. Some hospitals will provide patients with a special card to hand to the server to make it more discreet.

▶ **Boiled, broiled, steamed, poached, and grilled are safe bets, and ask twice about sauces.** Fried foods are off limits. Period. Make sure you verify that extra butter or oil is not put on your proteins during or after cooking. We know that eating moist food post-op is best tolerated, but in a restaurant most sauces are either high in fat (look for words like *cream, Alfredo, scampi,* *hollandaise*) or high in sugar (*sweet and sour, hoisin*) and should be avoided to prevent illness or consumption of extra calories. Broth-based sauces and marinaras are the safest bets.

▶ **Investigate ahead of time.** Before you dine out or eat at another person's home, get the menu ahead of time. Most restaurants make their menus available online. That way you know how to make a good choice upon arrival, or you can prepare a meal and eat *before* you go.

▶ **Order à la carte or bring something you can have.** It is likely you won't be able to eat more than a few bites of food, so try ordering just a plain chicken breast, shrimp cocktail, baked fish, or individual flatbread pizza with vegetable toppings. When dining at a friend's or family member's house, review your recipe collection (including this book) to find something that's a crowd pleaser and bring it for everyone to enjoy. That way, if you can't dine on the items your host serves, you'll know you have a safe item to fill you up.

▶ **Having good manners doesn't mean you have to overeat.** Order a to-go box immediately upon getting your food at the restaurant to avoid the server constantly asking if "something was wrong with the meal" as to why you didn't eat much—plus you don't want a huge plate of leftovers staring you in the face. At a friend's or family member's home, ask for a to-go plate if they insist you taste the leftovers or dessert. Then you can decide whether to throw it out once you get home, give it to someone else in the family, or eat it later. Being polite doesn't mean you have to stuff yourself with foods you can't eat or that will push you over your calorie limit.

Resources

Online Resources/Support Communities

Academy of Nutrition and Dietetics

www.eatright.org

The Academy of Nutrition and Dietetics, the largest organization of food and nutrition professionals in America, is a resource for finding credentialed experts in your area. Additionally, the Academy's website is a reference for reliable food and nutrition information founded in expert research.

American Society for Metabolic and Bariatric Surgery (ASMBS)

http://asmbs.org

ASMBS is the foremost organization in research for improving the treatment of obesity through surgical interventions. Check out this website to find a qualified surgeon in your area and learn more about the types of bariatric surgery. Additionally, ASMBS is a reference for reliable, evidenced-based facts about bariatric surgery and obesity treatment.

Bariatric Pal

www.bariatricpal.com

Founded by a bariatric surgery patient himself, Bariatric Pal is a social network for staying connected with other bariatric surgery information and fellow patients—both pre- and post-operatively. Access free forums and chat rooms that are specialized to each individual surgery type.

My Fitness Pal–Food and Activity Tracker

www.myfitnesspal.com

Use this free food and exercise tracker to monitor food intake and track activity to stay on target with your weight-loss regimen. You can closely monitor individual nutrients such as protein or sugars. There is also a recipe calculator for determining the nutrition information of your favorite homemade recipes. People who keep a journal or log of their food intake are more successful with weight loss than those who just follow a meal plan alone.

Obesity Action Coalition (OAC)

www.obesityaction.org

Check out this organization for reliable information about obesity treatment, educational resources, and connecting to local support and advocacy groups. Join the OAC to become a member of this community, which has a strong voice in the movement to both prevent and treat obesity as well as to fight obesity-related discrimination and weight bias.

The Obesity Society

www.obesity.org

The Obesity Society is an organization dedicated to studying obesity and its treatment. Reference this organization for reliable, up-to-date, evidenced-based information about obesity treatment. Find information here about educational programs and conferences around the country.

ObesityHelp

www.obesityhelp.com

An online support community for individuals and their families who struggle with obesity, ObesityHelp has a variety of resources for connecting with peers through support groups or forums. Forums are categorized based on a variety of topics, including ones on diseases related to obesity and type of bariatric surgery. Additionally, you can gain access to a wide variety of educational resources here.

References

Academy of Nutrition and Dietetics. "Bariatric Surgery." *Nutrition Care Manual,* July 1, 2016. www.nutritioncaremanual.org/about-ncm.

Aills, Linda, Jeanne Blankenship, Cynthia Buffington, Margaret Furtado, and Julie Parrott. "ASMBS Allied Health Nutritional Guidelines for the Surgical Weight Loss Patient." *Surgery for Obesity and Related Diseases* 4 (2008): S73–S108. doi:10.1016/j.soard.2008.03.002.

Centers for Disease Control and Prevention. "Adult Obesity Facts." Accessed September 24, 2016. www.cdc.gov/obesity/data/adult.html.

Cummings, Sue and Kellene A. Isom, eds. *Pocket Guide to Bariatric Surgery.* 2nd ed. Academy of Nutrition and Dietetics, 2015.

Mechanick, J. I., R. F. Kushner, H. J. Surgerman, J. M. Gonzalex-Campoy, M. L. Collazo-Clavell, A. F. Spitz, C. M. Apovian, et al. "American Association of Clinical Endocrinologists, the Obesity Society, and American Society for Metabolic and Bariatric Surgery Medical Guidelines for Clinical Practice for the Perioperative Nutritional, Metabolic, and Nonsurgical Support of the Bariatric Surgery Patient." *Obesity* 17, no. 51 (April 2009): S3–S72. doi:10.1038/oby.2009.28.

Mechanick, J. L., A. Youdim, D. B. Jones, W. T. Garvey, D. L. Hurley, M. M. McMahon, L. J. Heinbert, et al. "Clinical Practice Guidelines for the Perioperative, Nutritional, Metabolic and Nonsurgical Support of the Bariatric Surgery Patient—2013 Update:

Cosponsored by American Association of Clinical Endocrinologists, The Obesity Society, and American Society for Metabolic & Bariatric Surgery." *Obesity* 21, no. S1 (March 2013): S1–S27. doi: 0.1002/oby.20461.

Slade M. D., B. R. Levy, S. R. Kunkel, and S. V. Kasl. "Longevity Increased by Positive Self-Perceptions of Aging." *Journal of Personality and Social Psychology* 83, no. 2 (2002): 261–270. doi:10.1037//0022-3514.83.2.261.

Measurement Conversions

VOLUME EQUIVALENTS (DRY)

US STANDARD	METRIC (APPROXIMATE)
⅛ teaspoon	0.5 mL
¼ teaspoon	1 mL
½ teaspoon	2 mL
¾ teaspoon	4 mL
1 teaspoon	5 mL
1 tablespoon	15 mL
¼ cup	59 mL
⅓ cup	79 mL
½ cup	118 mL
⅔ cup	156 mL
¾ cup	177 mL
1 cup	235 mL
2 cups or 1 pint	475 mL
3 cups	700 mL
4 cups or 1 quart	1 L
½ gallon	2 L
1 gallon	4 L

VOLUME EQUIVALENTS (LIQUID)

US STANDARD	US STANDARD (OUNCES)	METRIC (APPROXIMATE)
2 tablespoons	1 fl. oz.	30 mL
¼ cup	2 fl. oz.	60 mL
½ cup	4 fl. oz.	120 mL
1 cup	8 fl. oz.	240 mL
1½ cups	12 fl. oz.	355 mL
2 cups or 1 pint	16 fl. oz.	475 mL
4 cups or 1 quart	32 fl. oz.	1 L
1 gallon	128 fl. oz.	4 L

OVEN TEMPERATURES

FAHRENHEIT (F)	CELSIUS (C) (APPROXIMATE)
250°F	120°C
300°F	150°C
325°F	165°C
350°F	180°C
375°F	190°C
400°F	200°C
425°F	220°C
450°F	230°C

Recipe Index

184

Index

Acknowledgments

Thank you to my sweet, loving, and caring husband, Christopher, for supporting my writing of this cookbook as well as all my endeavors in my career as a dietitian. And of course, for helping to "sample" all my recipes in addition to always being on "cleanup" duty.

To my entire family of talented chefs, especially my mom. You have inspired me to love food and cooking. You have shown me how to cook nutritious foods as a way of showing love for others. And with a grill master like my dad and chefs as talented as my three siblings and their spouses, a person is constantly compelled to keep making better and tastier recipes!

This book would not have been possible without the support of the comprehensive weight-loss team and bariatric surgery program I worked with for over seven years. Each and every one of the nurses, physicians, and administrative staff helped me learn about how to create a better experience for the patients undergoing bariatric surgery and help them achieve long-term weight-loss success. Especially Amy and Keri, who were always a short phone call away with a listening ear or expert advice.

To the late Dr. James Wallace, who was my mentor and the most talented general surgeon I have ever met. Thank you for teaching me everything I needed to know to help patients be successful after bariatric surgery.

I could not have written this book without inspiration from hundreds of patients seen in the Bariatric Surgery clinic at Froedtert Hospital. Each one of you inspired me every day to become a better dietitian, a more accomplished chef, and a more compassionate listener. Thank you for allowing me to be a part of your weight-loss journeys.

Finally, to the editing team at Callisto Media who helped me make this cookbook complete. I couldn't have done it without your support and guidance.

About the Author

SARAH KENT, MS, RDN, CD, is passionate about helping people overcome the barriers that prevent them from achieving their nutrition and weight-loss goals. For seven years, she served as lead dietitian for the bariatric surgery program at Froedtert & Medical College of Wisconsin, a nationally certified Center of Excellence for bariatric surgery. She offered a range of nutritional services to both pre- and post-operative bariatric patients and helped facilitate support groups. A Registered Dietitian Nutritionist with a master's degree in human nutrition, Sarah also earned a Certificate of Training in Adult Weight Management from the Academy of Nutrition and Dietetics. Currently, she is a senior dietitian and certified health and wellness coach at Froedtert Health. Sarah, her husband Chris, and their dog Ladis live in a suburb of Milwaukee, Wisconsin.

CPSIA information can be obtained
at www.ICGtesting.com
Printed in the USA
BVOW11s1657120117

473355BV00001B/1/P